Harrah
Christmas 2021

THE BOY WHO
LOST HIS SMILE

AUTHOR BIO

Lawrence Prestidge is an English author, actor and podcaster. Lawrence is best known for his popular children's novel *Terror at the Sweet Shop*. He has acted in some of the UK's biggest theatres and in Disneyland. His podcast *The Shapes of Stories* debuted during the lockdown of 2020 and has featured the likes of Gary Lineker, Eddie Izzard, Ann Widdecombe, Alastair Campbell, Sinitta, Rob Rinder, Ellie Simmonds MBE and other popular names.

This is Lawrence's first writing away from children's literature after wanting to support people who have wrestled with mental health struggles.

I wanted to write this to help people be less afraid. - Lawrence Prestidge

THE BOY WHO LOST HIS SMILE

LAWRENCE PRESTIDGE

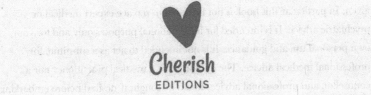

Cherish
EDITIONS

First published in Great Britain 2021 by Cherish Editions

Cherish Editions is a trading style of Shaw Callaghan Ltd & Shaw Callaghan 23 USA, INC.

The Foundation Centre

Navigation House, 48 Millgate, Newark

Nottinghamshire NG24 4TS UK

www.triggerhub.org

British Library Cataloguing in Publication Data

A CIP catalogue record for this book is available upon request from the British Library

ISBN: 978-1-913615-37-6

This book is also available in the following eBook formats:

ePUB: 978-1-913615-38-3

Lawrence Prestidge has asserted his right under the Copyright, Design and Patents Act 1988 to be identified as the author of this work

Cover design by More Visual

Typeset by Lapiz Digital Services

To my family and friends, who have endured the good, the bad and the ugly:

Thank you.

INTRODUCTION

I once met a guy who jumped off Waterloo Bridge and survived. He confessed to me, "Halfway down I thought it was a bad idea." But after battling with depression for many years, in that moment he decided that jumping was his only way out from the incredible pain he was experiencing. I wish I could say that I couldn't relate to this but I can. Not that I have ever jumped off Waterloo Bridge, but I do know the anguish that depression can bring.

My mental health crippled me for years; depression can be so debilitating that it's impossible to fully understand unless you've actually felt it. When I first experienced depression, I was terrified. I couldn't understand the overwhelming low feelings I was having; it was a strange pain I hadn't experienced before. You feel numb, weak and almost like you're in chains. Your joy has been robbed from you, and when you lose your joy, there comes a time where the blankness of the future is so extreme that the monstrosity of being alive can overwhelm you. It's awful to contemplate a futureless future. During my battle with depression and alcohol abuse, I really wish I'd known it was going to be okay in the end.

I believe that one of the most important things to realize about depression is that you're not alone. You won't be the first or last to go through it. Fortunately, it is becoming more acceptable to talk about mental illness, and it is being recognized for the disease it really is. But we need to acknowledge it and talk about it for that to continue to happen. I remember being so ashamed of talking about my depression that I kept it to myself for many years. That's partly because some people still think depression is the same as feeling down. There's still that attitude of, "What, you're depressed? Oh, just go and have a good walk, listen to some music and you'll be fine." Unfortunately, depression isn't like that. That's like saying, "Walk off the weather," but with depression, it's the weather inside you that's horrific and it's very real. Sadly, although people are starting to acknowledge depression more, some still suffer from a disease called "stigma". They find something unacceptable about depression so they brush it under the carpet. Telling a person with depression to "man up" is the equivalent of walking past someone sinking in quicksand and saying, "You're sinking. I'd try to avoid that if I were you."

There is a lot of confusion between depression and feeling sad, but sadness and depression are two very different things. Sadness is when something happens in your life and you temporarily feel unhappy about it. It can be fleeting or long-lasting and is a normal emotional reaction. Depression is a medical condition, an imbalance of chemicals in your brain that causes your worldview to become warped and stops you seeing things for what they really are.

I felt my depression grew when I was noticing how many incredible injustices there were in the world and what a mess we were making of things. I felt like screaming at happy people, "Guys, what are you not seeing?!" I almost felt like it was the happy people that needed medication! "You're feeling happy with how things are? You're mad!"

I began to drink alcohol to try to make myself happy, to be able to be sociable and to forget about my depression for a moment. But that was the worst thing I could do. Alcohol doesn't cheer you up, it reduces your inhibitions – it's a depressant that changes the balance of chemicals in your brain, altering the way you see and think things. So, my binge drinking only fuelled the depression, making it grow stronger and stronger.

I didn't drink alcohol every day but I certainly had a problem. If you're using alcohol as a coping mechanism for something, you may well have an alcohol problem that needs addressing. When I was binge drinking, I was violating my standards quicker than I could lower them – and that's a number one warning sign. But specific examples are often more telling, so if you recognize any of these situations, you have a problem, and the sooner you admit it, the better.

1 You're throwing up while pissing outside a Barclays doorway in the high street.
2 It's four o'clock in the morning and you decide that – regardless of how many drinks you've had that night – it's absolutely essential that you drive to the McDonald's drive-thru to get a Quarter Pounder with cheese.
3 You wake up in the morning next to someone and think, *Who the hell are you?*
4 You wake up alone and think, *Hey, someone's shit in my bed.*
5 You start drinking in London at lunchtime Saturday and when you have a comedown at three o'clock on Sunday afternoon, you pose the question, *Why am I in Belfast?*
6 And finally, you wake up on a Sunday morning and wonder why you have ordered two George Foreman grills, three packets of gummy bears, a Batman onesie and a life-size cardboard cut-out of Danny DeVito.

These were just some of the weekly occurrences for me and, to be honest, just the tip of a very large iceberg. I look back at my past and realize I had so many blackouts when I was drinking. The polite name for them is blackouts, but I feel like it's your conscience going into a witness protection program, saying to you as it exits swiftly:

"Lawrence, you're in a car with two strippers, a Polish drug dealer and some random-ass driver who is dropping off cocaine before you hope to get some action. I'm going now – good luck, I'll leave your penis on if you want, but I don't want any part of this."

I'm not proud of my behaviour from the ages of 18 to 25 at all. I look back with deep regret. I was so wrapped up in trying to feel good and be a fun person to be around that I didn't care how my actions hurt or affected other people. I didn't intentionally hurt anyone, especially my loved ones, but I was so immersed in my own shit that I was completely blind to the effect of my behaviour on others. Being that happy-go-lucky person was never really me. Looking back – because I didn't realize it at the time – I was putting on an act. As a kid, I was quite sweet and innocent; I had a performing arts background and loved the elementary things in life. I was happy. So much so that I remember going into my adolescence heartbroken – I didn't want to grow up and leave the things behind that I held dear: my love of Disney, reading and playing outside with my friends. I felt forced to let go before I was ready, trying to find a new identity that was more acceptable to the world as I got older. If I could talk to the teenage me, I would simply tell that kid to be himself. And as I got deeper and deeper into this dark, depressive hole, and was becoming more and more reliant on alcohol to try to be happy, I began to feel that life wasn't worth living.

In this book, I will be sharing my journey with you: the experiences and treatments I had, the medication I swallowed, the people I met and the time I spent in a mental health support centre. But there's one important aspect of how I changed my life that is, for me, a crucial part of giving you the full picture of my experiences, and that is my faith in God. I've not been a Christian my whole life; in fact when I left my Roman Catholic secondary school, I was pretty much done with any form of faith, religion or belief. So I can appreciate that some people are very reluctant to get into the whole "God" thing – and some will be rolling their eyes and sighing – but that's not a problem. This is my story, and God is part of it. You may have a different religion or belief system – Christian, Atheist, Buddhist, Muslim, Agnostic, Hindu, Scientologist, Jedi – or you may have none. It makes no difference. This isn't a book that's going to throw scripture and verses at you, pleading that you repent your sins. Everyone's faith and belief are their own personal decision. All I'm asking is for you to keep an open mind and let me share with you how my faith saved me.

At times, I used to sit back and wonder why depression is so widespread in today's society, and why suicide rates are skyrocketing, especially in younger people. In my opinion, there is something fundamental missing in the lives of many people and that is, simply, peace. We live in a society where social media dominates our lives. Everyone gets a running commentary of people's day-to-day experiences, each one setting up a comparison with others; and comparison is the thief of joy.

More and more people believe that their lives are validated by "likes" and approval from their peers and followers, as though popularity was the foundation of a happy life. But no amount of Instagram followers can fill a hole in your life, so these people are still left with this void. What is missing for them, I believe, is peace. You can never have peace if you're more interested in others liking you, than liking yourself. The greatest prison we live in is the fear of what other people think of us.

Experiencing inner peace for the first time was the biggest high in the world for me – better than any buzz that alcohol, drugs or sex could give me. It's something everyone should feel. This is the story of how I got there.

A disclosure though: this isn't a story where I simply "lived happily ever after" once I recovered from my main battle with depression. I'm still not sure if depression ever fully goes away; I keep the faith, and hope it will, and have felt it disappear in my life as I changed my lifestyle, so I hold onto that. But I must confess, during the Coronavirus pandemic I struggled with my mental health again. I wouldn't say it's ever been as bad as it was before, and that may be because I know how to help myself with it now, but it has certainly been tough. Like Covid-19, depression can take unpredictable directions. For some, it can be very mild for long periods, then quickly become severe. Some people may barely notice the effects of depression, while it pushes others to the extreme. During the pandemic, depression gathered and slowly started to overpower me again. If you give depression the slightest inroad, it will worm its way into your day-to-day life, growing stronger and stronger. I think I struggled during the pandemic for a few reasons, and that's because a lot of outlets that bring me joy were closed off to me: things like the gym, church, coffee shops, my work visiting schools, socializing with friends, and the theatre. I've really come to realize and appreciate just how much happiness these things bring me, drastically boosting my mental health. I never thought I was much of a "hugger", but I found myself actually longing for the day people when people felt comfortable enough to hug each other again. Having a hug and feeling that someone cares is a wonderful thing.

If you know someone battling any type of addiction or depression, my advice would be to listen and understand – not to try to fix it. Just as emotions wash over us, moods – good and bad – can do the same. At worst, suicidal thoughts can submerge us. If you know someone who is feeling that way, please be there for them. It is extremely important in making things better and keeping people safe until the peak of these thoughts passes. It will pass, it always does; people can endure the darkest moments. Sometimes the best treatment for people is just having someone to talk to.

Always hold onto that fundamental quality of faith: that no matter what pain you're going through currently, on the other side is something good. And no matter what, do not suffer in silence.

CONTENTS

CHAPTER 1

When talking about depression, I always felt that Robin Williams described it best in his portrayal of Genie in the 1992 movie *Aladdin*: "Phenomenal cosmic power – in an itty-bitty living space."

In a sense, we are all genies. We all have this amazing universal power in this teeny, tiny living space that we call a body. But depression has the ability to strip us of that power. It can destroy relationships, ruin the things that give us pleasure, disable our creativity and rob us of our peace and joy.

I remember when I had my first suicidal thought. It was the summer of 2014. I was lying in somebody else's bed, and I said to myself, "I don't want to do this anymore, I think I'm done."

Something inside me instantly spoke back: "Er, time out. Did you honestly just say you were done with life? You have a lot to be thankful for, you know. You have family and friends who love you, you've been lucky to live out some really cool experiences so far in life and you have so much to look forward to."

"I know," I replied to the voice, "but I'm tired of feeling like this."

"Okay, this is serious. I mean, what are you planning to do? Overdose? Throw yourself in front of a train?"

"No."

"Hang yourself?"

"Maybe."

"Okay, wow. This really has got out of hand. I feel like we've gone from mild depression to suicidal thoughts way too quickly. I mean, surely you couldn't go through with it anyway?"

"I don't know."

"Okay, okay, hold on. Let's stay calm and go over the facts. You've been drinking most of the night – is there any way that this may be influencing your thinking right now?"

"Maybe."

"Well, it's certainly something to think about. You're also in somebody else's bed – who's that in the bed there anyway?"

"I don't know."

"Well, don't discuss this with her. The last thing a girl wants to hear after a guy has slept with her is that they're depressed."

"Who am I talking to, anyway?"

"It's your conscience, dumbass," the voice replied.

Eventually shaking off that voice, I remember gingerly sneaking out of the girl's bedroom and walking home. It was about four in the morning and a three-mile walk, but I was hoping a long walk in the cold night air would clear my head of these bizarre suicidal thoughts that I was experiencing.

A few days later, I woke up feeling worse. The worst I had ever felt. My head felt like it was going to burst and my body like it was sinking. I not only woke up in my own urine – at least I think it was mine, I can't be certain, I hope it was – but I woke up to numerous voices whispering cruel things, filling my thoughts with a sense of hopelessness.

"What's the point anymore?"

"You're better off dead."

"You're going to feel like this forever."

"This is unfixable."

"There is only one way out."

As I got on with my Sunday, those voices and feelings of despair only intensified. I remember covering my face with a pillow just hoping for a moment of peace. I felt as though I was under attack from all directions but I was unable to move. I couldn't navigate the darkness around me, so I decided to stay right where I was and wallow in despair. *As much as it hurts, I'm just going to stay right here,* I thought to myself, *because this is what I deserve. I'm just a horrible person.*

But I couldn't stay where I was and let those feelings consume me, I needed to escape. I started going through my phone, messaging whoever I could to find someone to drag me away from this pit, someone who wouldn't ask for explanations.

An ex-girlfriend of mine was the first to respond. She thought it would be nice to catch up, and said to come over. I think I knew she still had feelings for me, which I didn't reciprocate, but I went anyway. I felt I had no choice. It was that or go insane. We shared a pizza and watched a movie. We had sex a couple of times.

Looking back, this was incredibly selfish of me. I didn't consider for a moment just how I might be making her feel; it was all about me. I was using the time with her as a distraction from my intense depression, without thinking that I was also giving her false hope that I may want us back together. I remember lying in bed with her and hearing the voices of hopelessness and despair creeping back into my head.

"I need to go," I said, as I slowly got out of bed to put on my clothes. As I got to my feet, I noticed a tear running down her face. I stopped what I was doing, my trousers hanging limply in my hand.

"What's wrong?" I asked. She turned her back on me and buried her face in the pillow.

"You got what you wanted and now you're just going. I probably won't hear anything from you for weeks – maybe even months," she said in a muffled and gloomy voice. Then her tone became angry. "You don't give a shit."

I didn't know what to say. I did care. I know I didn't want us back together, but I did feel genuinely awful for hurting her. My intense depression had taken over my life and made me feel out of control. Now it was stretching its tentacles further, causing me to make other people feel rubbish too.

"I'm sorry," I muttered. I didn't know what else to say. I could see that she was really upset, but I felt powerless to do anything about it. Staying would only reinforce the wrong impression and make the situation worse.

"I hate you," she said.

"Join the club," I muttered under my breath as I slithered out of her flat, genuinely despising myself for the way I had treated her, the way I had made her feel just to get a few hours out of the dark pit I was wallowing in.

"What a scumbag! What a selfish, fucking prick!" I shouted as I got into my car. What was I thinking? Was that worth it just to feel good for a couple of hours? Absolutely not.

I merged onto the motorway. Not only was I wrestling with a monstrous feeling of darkness inside me, I was also feeling a powerful sense of guilt. It began with how I had just treated my ex-girlfriend, but as I accelerated faster and faster down the motorway, I relived every mistake I had ever made, saw the faces of everyone I had hurt along the way – family, friends, ex-girlfriends, the driver of the slow-moving car in front of me the other week who I swore at as I overtook. I was regretting anything and everything I could.

"Just do it. Just end it all," a voice hissed. "Just make the pain go away." It felt like a group of terrorists was gagging my conscience to prevent it from screaming, "Don't do it, Lawrence!"

"The motorway is clear, just drive yourself off it as fast as you can. It'll be over with quickly," the sinuous voice continued.

I was in the fast lane, foot flat on the floor. It was as if something else was in complete control of my body. I was on auto-pilot. It was time to do it. I thought of my friends and family, praying they would forgive me. I closed my eyes, hoping that the whole experience would be as quick and painless as possible. Then, for a split second, I opened my eyes to see a blue van directly in front of me. A collision was inevitable. My instincts kicked in and I slammed my foot on the brake, but I was too close. I rear-ended the vehicle with a sickening thud, lurched forward then was flung back into my seat.

I must have blacked out for a few moments, but couldn't have been out too long. As I started to come to, both the van driver and the passenger were climbing out of their cab. I breathed a sigh of relief, thankful that no one seemed seriously hurt. But relief soon turned to panic as I watched two stocky young men approaching my car. My first thought was, *Shit! They're not going to be happy with me one bit. I'm going to get my ass kicked.*

The driver of the blue van opened my door. I held my breath, expecting a tirade of abuse.

"Are you all right, mate?" came his concerned voice.

I was totally taken aback. His face was serious, he looked as though he worked out, and I had just put a huge dent in the back of this guy's van. The best scenario I imagined was being called every name under the sun.

"I think so," I replied, slowly climbing out of the car. Luckily, it was around two in the morning, and the motorway was more or less clear.

"What happened?" the other lad asked me. I took a deep breath. *Now I need an explanation and quick*, I thought. Luckily this is where the skills I picked up in acting and improvisation came in handy.

"You know, I've been ill for a few days and I must have dozed off. I'm so sorry, boys, are you both okay?" I asked.

They assured me they were both fine. There was actually more damage to my car than to their van. We took photos of our vehicles and exchanged insurance details. They were concerned for my wellbeing and wanted to make sure I was well enough to continue with my journey. They even checked my car for me to make sure it was safe to drive. After I assured them I was okay, I wished them well and we both drove away. I sat back, completely stunned; did I just come close to taking my own life?

The next few days were a bit of a blur. I was on a summer break from working at a school, and spent most of the time staying at home during the day and hitting bars and clubs at the weekend. I was trying to shelter myself from any other opportunities to take my own life. I was more or less living in my PJs.

As I lay on the sofa watching the news on television one night, a story broke that stopped my breath for a second, then stopped my life dead in its tracks and turned it right around.

"We have just got word that the Academy Award-winning actor and comedian Robin Williams has died," the announcer said. "Reports suggest this was an apparent suicide by hanging."

CHAPTER 2

Sometimes I look back and try to put my finger on exactly where my mental health problems may have started, and I think it was during my time at secondary school. I remember there being this moment where I had a sudden realization that life could sometimes be very cruel and unjust, or simply not make much sense.

At 14 I had just recently lost one of my best friends. Tom had died in a road traffic accident on his way home from school. Tom and I always walked to the bus stop together, and I can still vividly see him getting on the bus that he would sadly never get off. Trying to get my head around death at that time, under those circumstances, was something I really struggled with. It was my first experience of death; all my grandparents were still alive, and I had never had to deal with any type of family bereavement. Now, one of my best friends, just 14 years old, had his life snatched away in the blink of an eye. I searched for an explanation but couldn't come up with anything. There was no justice in what happened to Tom.

Our Roman Catholic school tried to help Tom's friends as best they could. They wanted to assure us that there was no reason to be upset, and that Tom was now at peace and with God. The day after he died, we had a huge mass for Tom at the school with a big memorial and a huge picture of him on display. I understand what the school was trying to do, but it was all a bit overwhelming. They offered us some counselling, but at that age, I found it hard to share my feelings with a stranger. His other friends may have felt differently – some of them perhaps were used to Catholic mass more than I was and found it completely normal. But I was devastated. In 24 hours, not only had I lost one of my best friends, but I had also lost my faith in God, and I was grieving for that, too. Why would God allow someone like Tom to die at such a young age? It just didn't make any sense to me.

God can't be real, I kept thinking to myself. *What kind of God would let this happen?* I'm not sure I truly believed in God again for another ten years. Not fully, anyway. My school friends are now all atheists.

My best friend gone and my faith undermined, the adolescent struggle to find my identity was a tough one for me. I didn't really know who I was. I wanted to fit in with my peers, but I was nowhere near ready to give up my childhood and the innocent games I still loved. It seemed as though I had to choose between being teased relentlessly by my so-called friends and giving up everything that made me who I was.

When young people are asked to list the first words that come to mind when they think of men, they usually come up with terms like "brave", "strong" or "fearless". When it comes to asking them to describe women, they'll usually say "kind", "gentle" and "caring". It's important for us to ask how and why we automatically use these stereotypes. Where might young boys get the mentality that it's weak for men to cry? Or even that men are strong and women are weak?

It's important for men to have the opportunity to talk to each other about this, and I believe through conversations with each other we will see that these thoughts are usually influenced by our society. Toxic masculinity is defined as a set of negative behaviours that men believe they have to follow in order to be "proper men".

To me, this pressure put on young males today to conform to outdated ideas of masculinity is outright frightening. And it results in boys today having difficultly expressing their emotions, accepting emotional vulnerability or admitting to any sadness or weakness. I know that happened to me. My young adult life was a lie. When I felt at my weakest, I pretended to be strong. When I was feeling insecure, I pretended to be confident. For a massive portion of my life, I put on a show for other people that made me gradually lose any sense of who I really was. It was exhausting trying to be "man enough" to be accepted by everyone until, when I eventually got to a point when I was tired of performing, I wasn't sure of my identity anymore.

All I wanted was to be accepted and liked by the other boys. To do that, I had to embrace what they defined as masculine and reject the feminine, or face rejection myself. The concept that men are strong and women are weak is wrong – it's toxic and it has to end.

It took me to the age of nearly 30 years old to realize that I didn't like who I was as a person. I had conflict within myself and conflict with the world that told me who I should be as a man. A lot of this resulted from throwing away innate qualities because they were considered "feminine". But is a man who's loving, kind, sensitive, nurturing and expressive really so wrong?

My resentment spilled over in my attitude toward my parents. I felt they had brought me up to be too soft, too oversensitive. I felt like my Dad never taught me how to do "manly" things like fishing, how to fight, DIY and other "man stuff". Instead, they taught me what they knew. They taught me about being kind, how to express myself and work hard.

I can't help but wonder why men feel like they can't tell each other they're hurting. In my experience, it just doesn't happen. We can talk about sports, politics and women, but that's about as far as male conversation goes. If it comes to talking about our feelings, our fears and our pain, it's almost like we've crossed a forbidden line. Men worry that just discussing these things, even to their closest male friends, might be portrayed as weak.

We need to redefine what toughness, bravery and strength mean, as men. Can we not use these qualities to explore our hearts? In my opinion, the toughest, bravest and strongest thing you can do is talk about your feelings – especially when you are not okay. Men shouldn't need permission to express themselves.

Sometimes, I look at children and worry they are losing that sense of innocence and imagination far too early. We can see the wonder in their play and the beauty in their smiles and the innocence in their hearts. But on the flip side, there is too much exposure to indecent images, graphic video games and antisocial behaviour at such a young age. I feel we must celebrate the positive and encourage children to live in a world of imagination. They have plenty of time to step into our adult world and experience its harsh reality – let them live in the world of imagination while they have the chance.

Let's encourage sensitivity and not force children to hide their sensitive side in order to fit in, as I did. I think there is a misconception that sensitive people are weak and fragile and that you have to treat them cautiously, as though you are walking on eggshells. That's not the case. Sensitive souls just have their senses on high alert, their emotions magnified. What you might experience as a passing sadness, for them would be a deep despair; your happiness could be a feeling of pure ecstasy for them. It's weird – sometimes when I hear some very sad news, I don't react much, but then feel myself shedding tears over the movie *Dumbo*. I even remember as a kid watching the movie *Jaws* for the first time. It had so much of an effect on me that I didn't go in the sea for several years. Even now, I make sure that if I am in the sea there are a few people further out than me so that I have a bit of a warning to get out quickly! But that's no reason why I should endure comments like, "you're too sensitive", "you always take things to heart" or, "oh, it's just a joke, man up".

These are the earliest memories I have of feeling as though the world was in fact a very dark place, and the first time I felt a very real, different type of sadness – which I now know to be depression.

Thankfully, getting involved in theatre and acting kept me somewhat stable, offering me an escape. But I was slowly creating a persona that I felt would be more acceptable to others as I got older – the person I thought everyone else wanted me to be. As the years went on, the more I tried putting on this act for everyone else, the more it threatened to cause me to self-destruct.

CHAPTER 3

Hearing the news of Robin Williams' death devastated me emotionally. I felt such an intense and personal grief. It's weird, isn't it? Someone that you've never met can have such a huge impact on your own life. It always feels sad when a celebrity dies because we feel as though we know them – and it reminds us that no one is immortal. We remember how we felt when the tragedy of Amy Winehouse hit the news, how the world mourned for Princess Di, the sad death of Caroline Flack, and perhaps even where we were when we found out Michael Jackson had died. We listen to other celebrities who pay their tributes on social media, and we post our own messages of sympathy.

There was a variety of reasons why the death of Robin Williams really hit me hard. One was the fact that I felt as though I had grown up with him: from discovering him as Genie in *Aladdin*, to seeing him star in *Hook*, *Jumanji* and *Mrs Doubtfire*, then, as I got older, admiring his raw acting ability in roles such as his Academy Award-winning performance in *Good Will Hunting*, *Patch Adams*, *One Hour Photo* and *Good Morning, Vietnam*. After my short acting career, it was his film *Dead Poets Society* that had inspired me to get a job in education. I found his fast-paced humour, improvisation and sheer acting ability absolutely mesmerizing.

Robin Williams was someone who brought people so much laughter and joy. He was arguably the funniest person in the world, yet someone who was in so much pain. I remember thinking that if someone like Robin Williams can make the decision to take his own life, is anyone truly safe? Is depression a death sentence?

I recently heard a heartbreaking story about Robin Williams from a London theatre director I know well. He told me he had met Robin at a fundraising event where Robin performed a short stand-up routine unannounced. It was a special surprise at the end of the night. The audience were howling with laughter; he had stolen the show.

At the end of the performance, this director said to Robin, "Thank you so much for coming tonight. That was something special. Bloody brilliant. I haven't seen so many people laughing so much."

Robin replied, "Well, that's good, because I feel like shit."

The director had told me he laughed at Robin's response. He said Williams even delivered that line as if he was joking, like it was a line from his act. But did it have a deeper meaning? Was it a cry for help? I know it's something that haunts the director to this day.

The day after Robin Williams died, I rang up the doctor's surgery and made an appointment to see a GP.

I'm not going to let this mental health problem take me, I remember thinking to myself. However, in the days leading up to my appointment, I tried talking myself out of attending. I was looking for a reason to cancel the appointment. *Today's been okay*, I'd tell myself. *Perhaps I'm over the worst of it.*

It's important not to be fooled by these thoughts. Treat depression as a person – a really malicious, horrible person. Depression is sinister, it lies to you, manipulates you and plays cruel tricks on you. It will completely overpower you one day, back off another day and linger in wait for the perfect opportunity to cause as much damage as possible.

One of the biggest hurdles in battling depression is accepting you have it and are willing to admit it to someone. It's a dark, cruel, surreal bubble. But you must hold on to the fact that you know that is not true and that if you find the courage to reach out and get help, it will be a game changer.

So I managed to get myself to the doctor and was sitting in the waiting room. I felt terribly anxious. Every fibre of my being was telling me to run away.

There's no way I'm going to be able to actually admit what's wrong with me. This was a bad idea, I remember thinking to myself. I was trying to think of other reasons I could perhaps tell the doctor why I'd come. Anything but the truth.

Maybe I could say I'm just having a few problems sleeping recently? Shall I just say I have a fever? Is Ebola still a thing? Thoughts raced through my head.

"Lawrence Prestidge," I heard a voice say.

Dr Galt was her name, an amazing doctor – I can't speak highly enough of her. I approached her office, completely convinced I would bottle it and not to tell her what was really wrong with me. I would just make something up on the spot. I sat down; my heart felt like it was beating at 100 miles per hour. I had never really understood people who got so anxious that they began to sweat. I did then – it was happening to me. I felt sweat streaming down my spine.

"So how can I help?" Dr Galt asked.

My rehearsed lie was on the tip of my tongue. It was locked and loaded and ready to shoot out, but something was holding me back. I noticed that Dr Galt was making very strong eye contact with me. She was ready to listen to every word I had to say. I could feel it.

Maybe I can actually trust her with this, I thought. *Maybe she won't judge me, and she'll actually understand. She might just be able to help me beat this awful dark feeling that's consuming me.*

"I've not been feeling great lately," I remember saying. It almost felt like a hiccup. It even caught me off guard as I said it – the admission just slipped out.

Once I had said this, I was able to express everything. It was as if a flood of water had broken free from the dam that had been confining it for so long. I was able to let my feelings and emotions flow. I told her everything: how low I was feeling, the suicidal thoughts that had become more and more real and regular, my binge drinking. It felt as though I had been pinned down and the bonds were suddenly cut. Dr Galt didn't say a word whilst I spoke. She just sat and listened, not interrupting me once. Her strong eye contact never faltered.

She seemed warm and personable. I felt like I could trust her. As I finished talking, a few tears ran down my face. I had done it. I had said it all.

There were a few seconds of silence before Dr Galt handed me a tissue and said, "Lawrence, it's going to be okay. I'm going to help you."

Just hearing that itself was a huge, almost palpable relief and soothed my cloudy head. My hands stopped shaking and my shoulders slumped down. I took a long, deep breath. I felt as though I had taken my first major step on my journey to recovery. I felt almost proud.

CHAPTER 4

Dr Galt prescribed some medication and made me another appointment for a week's time. I would see her every week. She encouraged me to explain the situation to work and tell them what I was going through. That took some courage but the human resource lady was amazing, so I went back to work. Unfortunately, not everyone was so understanding. When word got around the school that I was struggling with depression, I was disappointed to find that things became really difficult. I was even teased by some of the staff – maybe they saw it as banter, I'm not really sure. I didn't find it funny anyway. It made me feel embarrassed, weak and a failure.

My line manager was one of those who was not very supportive. She gave the distinct impression that she suspected I was using the depression as an excuse to be off work. It didn't help that she was aware that I continued to binge drink at the weekends. I'd bump into teachers now and again whilst I was off work and getting drunk on a Saturday night, so I imagine this got back to her. Her attitude changed our working relationship completely, as it was clear she wanted me out. Maybe she had a point, I don't know. I could see how it might look but I couldn't convince her that my depression was real. I would have loved the constant despair I was feeling to have been nothing more than a creative hoax to get some time off, but sadly it was only too real and affecting me every day.

I loved my job at the school, working with some of the vulnerable students and those with behaviour problems, and also teaching drama, because of my experience in acting. But working at a school is one of the most difficult environments when you are depressed. You are responsible for big groups of people, which in itself can be stressful and demanding. I didn't have the energy required anymore and didn't feel supported by them. I could no longer give my best when I felt emotionally, mentally and physically exhausted.

The medication I was on took a little while to kick in, but when it did I noticed small, positive changes. My sleep pattern was better, I had motivation to go to the gym, I was eating better and I was even able to get joy out of the little things in life – just popping to the coffee shop, watching the football and reading. I had a couple of months of feeling okay. I wouldn't say the depression had gone but it almost felt like it had shrunk. The overwhelming, dark despair that was on top of me, was now a little bouncy ball that I could hide away in my pocket.

It's important not to think that any form of medication is just going to instantly save you and make things okay again. There is no magic pill. You do still experience really bad days, and when you are experiencing one of these bad days and feel like you're unable to leave the house or your bed, it can be painfully difficult. But remembering the very worst days of my depression helped me get through the others. "I've got through worse," I'd often tell myself. "Tomorrow is going to be a better day." Say these things out loud!

CHAPTER 5

Another thing depression brings with it into your life is an ability to deceive.

I was going to bed every night thinking to myself, *What now, huh? Where the fuck do I go from here? Every day just gets harder and harder, and I'm so over fighting this right now.* Just having thoughts of contemplating suicide is soul-destroying – going to bed each night with the hope you don't wake up to face the pain.

At the same time, I wasn't being honest about it. I felt as though depression made me into a master of lying and deceit. People who loved me and cared for me would ask, "Is everything okay?" "Where are you going?" "Do you want to talk?" For whatever reason, I couldn't open up to them. It felt easier to lie than put the burden onto someone I loved. Whether it was my family, closest friends or people I trusted, my answers would always be: "I'm fine." "I'm just going to see a friend." "Talk about what? Honestly, everything is fine."

In reality, I wasn't fine at all. I was usually going out to try and clear my head from the awful feelings I was having, and I needed to talk to someone more than anything.

When I look at photos of myself on social media, I see a guy with his friends, seemingly having a good time, smiling as if I was without a care in the world. I find it very hard to look at those pictures. In fact, I've deleted many of them. All I see now is someone putting on an act. I may have been smiling and looking like I was having a fabulous time, but in reality, I was in the most pain I had ever been in my life, desperately confused and screaming for help on the inside.

I really can't express how important it is to open up about depression. I find the more you hide those painful moments, the more likely suicide will happen. I can honestly say, the moments when I've been holding in my pain the most are always the points when I've come closest to considering taking my own life.

If you're ever feeling like the monstrosity of life is too much to bear and you feel you've started to contemplate suicide, please reach out to a loved one immediately. I know it's easier said than done but it will save your life. Please just reach out to someone. Call a friend, partner, doctor or family member and let them know how you're feeling. Finding that connection, that love, overpowers the suicidal thoughts. I used to think it wasn't okay to tell people that I needed help and that I was struggling, but I now know that it's not just okay, it's absolutely the right thing to do – don't let depression lie to you and tell you it isn't.

There are things I'm still working on, of course. I used to be notorious among my friends for pushing people away. Whether it was girlfriends, friends or some family members, it felt easier to push them away from my weird, very dark world. I didn't want any of them to even come close to feeling that sinister, depressive energy. It didn't seem fair to bring people into that space. Although it's something I've improved on, it's also still something that's a work in progress. I'm very careful about who I let into my little, weird bubble.

I have made several suicide plans over the years. I've written letters to loved ones ready for them to find. I've written lists of things to do before going through with it, thought about dates that would cause the least disruption for my family. I even remember feeling relief and excitement at the prospect of the pain soon being over when a date was in sight. I was going to be done suffering, I was going to be done with the struggle, I was going to be done with the confusion, I was going to be done with my mistakes – it was all going to be gone.

I used to fantasize about how I'd do it. Every so often, the urge would come. When a train would be approaching on a station platform, a little voice would whisper, "Jump." Driving late at night on a clear road going 90 miles per hour. Seeing how long I could last holding my breath in the bath, how long the sensation of feeling breathless would last before becoming too much to bear.

When depression was at its worst for me, I felt dead inside. I felt like a zombie. In a way, feeling like I was already dead brought me a step closer to physically dying. Suicide felt like the next logical step.

When I was convinced I was not far away from taking my own life, I started to take a moment to look at things for what I thought would be the last time. I remember when I was convinced I was having my last Christmas and feeling like I was seeing certain friends for the last time. I made sure I told them I loved them in those moments. I remember thinking it would be the last time I would walk past a certain building, and even more horrific, the last time I would ever have a Domino's pizza. I remember thinking I was watching my last Newcastle game on television. They lost. *Useless bastards couldn't even see me off with a win*, I thought to myself.

During what I felt were going to be my final days, I decided I wanted to have sex one last time. But at the same time, I didn't want to put any ex-girlfriends or lovers of mine through any stress or sadness when I had taken my life only days later. I was very aware of not wanting to make anyone feel shit just to fulfil a desire for the final time. I just wanted no-strings-attached, no-questions-asked, sex.

The best way for me to do that was to start looking up escorts online. I wanted to find a stunning escort I could just have my last hurrah with.

I noticed one person's advert. *Pretty hot!* I remember thinking to myself. She lived fairly local as well. I could probably drive to hers in about 45 minutes. Destiny it said her name was – I have to say, I wasn't convinced that was her real name at all. But I didn't care, she could say her name was Ernie for all I cared at that point.

I gave a fake name myself, surprised by how long I spent debating what I'd like to be called. I went with James in the end, not exactly original I know, but there was almost a James Bond feel to me going undercover.

I remember driving to Destiny's house, feeling rather excited. *I'm going to make sure this is the best sex I've ever had*, I thought to myself. I parked up and knocked on her door. I remember she took a minute or two to answer. I wanted her to hurry up. I didn't really want her whole street seeing me, as I imagined they might often see men coming and going from the house. I didn't really want it to get out that this was on my to-do list before ending my life. I'm not too sure why I cared so much. I think I just wanted to make sure this experience was as private as possible. I just wanted to get it out of my system and go. She opened the door. At first, I remember feeling relief that she was as attractive as she looked in her photos. She had a hoodie on but was showing lots of cleavage, with the hoodie only half zipped up. *Gentlemen, start your engines*, I remember thinking to myself.

"Hi, handsome," she greeted. "Come on in."

"Hi! How's your day been? Been busy?" What a stupid question to ask! She's an escort, not a fucking cab driver. No wonder she ignored the question.

As I walked in, something pretty strange happened to me. I started to shake, I wasn't really in control of my speech, and most tragically my penis seemed to have stage fright. I had travelled to her house and waltzed in all confidently, trying to act like Mr Big Shot, but the act I was putting on soon started to crack as I sat on her sofa. My bloody conscience started piping up at me:

"So, is this really going to make you feel better?"

The more I asked myself that question, the more I realized it wouldn't. I'm sure it would have felt great for a short period of time but would undoubtedly have made me feel awful long term.

"You've not done this before have you?" Destiny sat next to me and started to stroke my arm. She took off her hoodie so she was only sat in her erotic lingerie.

"Is it that obvious?" I sighed.

"There's no need to be nervous, sweetie," she said as she started to kiss my neck. "Do you want to go upstairs? I'll be gentle if you want me to."

"Maybe a drink first?" The reality of the situation was starting to dawn on me.

She stopped kissing me and took a step back. "Babe, why did you come here?" she asked me.

"Well, not to have my eyes tested." She looked at me; she didn't laugh. "I'm sorry, I've just never done this before."

"Look, let's not waste each other's time, babe. If you've gone off this, don't worry, I won't charge you. I'm not too sure why you're even here to be honest."

"What do you mean?"

"Let's just say you seem a lot different to my other clients – and don't worry, I mean in a good way," she answered as she stroked my arm with a smile. At the time it seemed a little condescending, like I was being a nice, polite little boy.

"What makes you think I'd come here if I didn't want to?" I asked. She was right, of course, but I was curious.

"You're acting like a gentleman. At the door you greeted me, asked how my day was and smiled. Last night I had a client whose first question to me as I opened the door was, 'How much more do I need to give you for anal?'"

"Well, that might have been my next question," I joked.

"Also, the fact you're shaking like a leaf kind of makes me feel like you're in two minds about this. Usually, guys come here and can't get their clothes off quick enough – it's like they're competing against the countdown clock. Especially if they just book in for 15 minutes with me, that's always a barrel of laughs."

I felt myself go red-faced. "I feel bad for wasting your time."

"Don't worry, babe. I'm in my home, glass of red on the go. Trust me, you haven't messed me around too much. If I had driven to yours and this happened, I probably wouldn't be impressed!" She smiled. "Go home, get a McDonald's and grab a beer and chill.

Whatever it is you're going through, or whatever her name is that's making you feel so crap, this isn't the answer. It's her loss. Trust me," she said with a wink.

I didn't comment at that remark. *I wish I was just rebounding over a girl*, I thought to myself.

I remember walking out of Destiny's house and, however strange it seems – and it seemed strange to me – I couldn't help but smile as she closed the door.

"Fucking hell, even the hooker feels sorry for me," I sighed.

CHAPTER 6

There is one thing I can't stress enough that you must not do when you are going through depression and that's drink. Sadly, I learnt that lesson the hard way.

After a few weeks of feeling okay, I started to go out, and was drinking a lot more – against the advice of my doctor. I felt like it was okay because I was in control of my depression.

I can handle it now. I've got this, I would think to myself. Boy, was I wrong.

I almost feel like depression had a plan to get me drinking again. I was starting to win the battle and it needed a game plan.

"Well, today's not been the best day, maybe now you've had a break from drinking just one or two wouldn't hurt to give you a little buzz? You've done the hard bit now. You're in control," depression would whisper to me.

Before I knew it, I was binge drinking every weekend again, having lots of casual sex with whoever I'd met in nightclubs, getting a short-term buzz to feel good for a very short periods of time. The comedown was horrific. My weekends were spent fuelling the depression to come back stronger and stronger.

Remember alcohol is a depressant: it can blunt your immune system, and is simply bad news for people who struggle with anxiety and depression. If you're going through a tough time and are still drinking heavily at the weekends, it may be worth asking whether you would benefit from letting that go, because perhaps it's preventing your recovery. It's worth examining your relationship with alcohol to establish whether it is making things harder for you. I mean, by all means, do whatever it is that makes you happy, but isn't that the keyword there? "Happy"? Is your relationship with alcohol a pure one, or is it a riddled, dark relationship? Is it holding you back?

Sadly, alcohol and suicides almost go hand in hand. More than one-third of suicide victims drink just before their death. I believe that's because alcohol and depression combined makes us lose all sense of rational thought.

It's hard to say whether alcohol causes depression or depression causes alcohol. I think both are true for different people. For me, realizing alcohol could give me a short-term release from depression for a few hours led to an alcohol dependency at weekends, just so I'd not seem miserable when I was out with my friends. A lot of people believe that it not only enables you to have a good time, but it also reduces the physical feeling of sadness. If you've ever had a drink just to help you escape from sadness, then you know it doesn't help for very long at all.

Alcohol is a weapon, a tool depression uses to drag people into its pit. It's deceptive: it gives a short-term buzz but the comedown we can experience is horrific. By using alcohol to numb your sadness, you're also numbing your joy. When you're using alcohol to self-medicate and escape the pain of depression, it just allows the depression to grow stronger and last longer. The more you use alcohol as a tool to numb the depressive feelings, the more alcohol you will need next time to reach the same temporary relief.

If I could still binge drink and feel I could easily overcome depression and anxiety from overwhelming me, I'm sure I would. But I can't. That's a fact I eventually had to swallow.

I'm not trying to convince you to stop drinking; I still drink a small amount. But I did need to spend nearly a year sober and get help before I could allow alcohol back into my life in a healthy way. If you feel like you are in control and you can handle the backlash, and it's totally worth it, then good for you. Only you know what's best for you; only you can be real with yourself.

I can only tell you my opinion from my experiences. I'm not an expert on alcoholism or mental health, but I am an expert on my own story. I was there when it happened. Well, I was present anyway.

Looking back, I was certainly struggling far more with my depression when I was binge drinking than I ever was when I wasn't. At the time, I didn't know that by drinking I was making things worse. I was mixing antidepressants, sleeping medications and painkillers with alcohol. I'm sure I don't need to tell you that's not a good mix! But I was desperate and addicted to having that short-term relief from depression. By mixing all of this with large amounts of alcohol, I made my antidepressants ineffective and the depressive feelings more intense.

Drinking whilst going through depression is kind of like being an out-of-shape footballer … technically you can play, just not as well as the others. And it's not a nice experience for anyone involved.

After a couple of months of binge drinking at the weekends, sleeping around and spending money I didn't have, I was back to square one.

It was early November. I woke up one morning and thought, *Y'know what, I can't do this anymore. I'm going to kill myself today. I'm going to do it TODAY!* I even remember having a short buzz of excitement that this would be the last day of feeling like this.

I was alone in my house and had the perfect opportunity to do it. I planned to hang myself. I was going to do it using a wardrobe and a belt. I even took a towel and put it between my neck and the belt. I got as far as securing the belt around my neck, with the other end of the belt attached to a wardrobe railing, and the belt wedged between the closed wardrobe door and door frame. I had written a letter to my family; it must have been about ten pages long or so. I gave them messages for my close friends. I wanted to reassure them there was nothing they could have done to stop this, and tried to explain the enormous amounts of pain I was feeling daily.

I was in position, all I had to do now was do it. But I was frozen in that moment. All the awful voices that had been continually whispering to me, encouraging me to take my own life everyday were now silent. They were now watching me, on the edge of their seats, waiting for me to do it. It was like they had dragged me to the edge of a cliff and were all watching and waiting for me to jump. As much as these voices had been egging me on to take the plunge, when it came down to that decisive moment, it was all on me.

I didn't really have much faith at this point. But I wanted to pray, just in case.

"God, if you're there. Please just understand the pain I'm going through. I'm tired of fighting this. Please forgive me," I muttered.

As I closed my eyes ready to take the lunge forward, I felt a voice, a feeling in my heart, one I had never felt before.

"Please, don't do this, Lawrence. You are loved. I have a plan for you. Trust in me. Please don't do this," I kept hearing repeatedly.

I remember trying to figure out just who I was hearing. Was it my conscience? Whatever it was, its presence was overwhelming – a sense of unconditional love I don't think I've ever felt before. I detached myself from the belt and threw it against the wall. I collapsed on the floor and leant against the wardrobe, sobbing.

Looking back, it's a terrifying thing to think about. If I had kept up the binge drinking to the same extent, I really don't think I would be here now.

CHAPTER 7

Soon after was an experience that changed my life forever. I would chance upon my first real encounter with what I believe was Jesus. I was still binge drinking at the weekends and this particular weekend I had gone to Bedford, which is where I went to university. That night, I had got very drunk again. I can't remember too much about the night itself, but I can clearly remember how it ended. But during the night I had met a girl in the nightclub, and we were obviously getting on well, drinking and dancing together. She told me she was single. As we left the club together to get some food, three guys approached us on Bedford high street.

"What's going on here then?" one of them said.

"What are you on about?" I replied.

I could see the look of dread on the girl's face. She looked like she had seen a ghost.

"What are you doing with my missus?" he asked, with his two friends either side of him.

"I thought you were single?" I said to the girl.

"I am, we broke up recently. He just can't accept it," she replied.

"How recently is this?" I asked.

"Last night," she answered, as if that was completely justified.

"Well, thanks for the fucking heads up ..." I said to her.

"Look, mate, I'm not really sure what's going on here between the two of you, but ..." I didn't say any more as the three of them began to lay into me. I had been punched on a couple of different occasions by disgruntled boyfriends, though luckily, I hadn't been hurt too much before. But this was more serious. Fists were flying at my head – there could only have been six but it felt like a hundred. I covered my face, trying to protect myself as much as I could. Kicks and knees were now starting to make their way up to my face too. It's almost too hard to say how long this went on for. It all seemed in slow motion. What seemed a ten-minute attack on me, probably was only about 30 seconds or so.

It got to the point where I didn't care anymore. Although I was instinctively trying to protect my face and my head, I remember being resigned to being killed. I was hoping they were going to kill me. I was ready to die. *Come on then you fuckers, kill me,* I remember thinking to myself. *Just do it.*

This was the point where something amazing happened to me. I remember it so clearly. As I was being attacked, I had a surreal out-of-body experience. I was above my body, watching it all happen in slow motion. I remember wanting to run back to my body. I was thinking, *Wait, if I'm watching this then who is controlling my body?* But all that worry and panic almost instantly went away. As I looked at myself, I felt an overwhelming sense of peace. I wish I could describe it to you in more detail and explain how amazing this feeling was but I can't. It's something you just have to feel for yourself. I didn't want that feeling to end.

All my teenage and young adult life, I had been wanting to find happiness and something to fulfil me, whether that was searching for fame, love, popularity, attention, sex or alcohol. I realized I had been searching in all the wrong places. What I needed to find was peace within myself.

The feeling I had was overwhelming. I wish I could feel like that for every second of every day for the rest of my life. It was as if I knew Jesus was there, protecting me.

I felt absolutely no pain whatsoever. I just had this overwhelming sense of peace. I then started to hear a soothing, loving voice, instructing me to forgive these people. Although what was happening to me was really traumatic, I was feeling an overpowering sense of forgiveness towards my assailants. I noticed people gathering around, pushing the attackers off me as I lay on the floor.

But at that moment, nothing really mattered to me. I was at peace and I was safe. At this point, I knew without a doubt there was far more to life as we know it. There is something out there, something spiritual. I knew there was something after death; we do have a creator of some kind. I respect everyone's beliefs and their faith, but I honestly struggle to understand people who think we are all here by accident; I know there is something else. It's up to each of us to draw our own conclusions.

CHAPTER 8

As Henry David Thoreau said, "Never look back unless you're planning to go that way."

This is how people get trapped; it's how depression traps you. There's something inevitable about the way depression works. It's going to try and draw you backwards. It's going to try and get you to focus on the bad things that have happened. It wants you to see your mistakes; it wants you to wallow in your mistakes. Your energy is always going to go where your attention is, and if your attention is on the past, then that's where you're going to spend your time and you're never going to be able to look ahead to the future.

You can't allow your mistakes to continuously torment you. You're never going to become the person you're capable of becoming until you can forgive yourself. You would never allow a thief to run into your home and live there rent-free, so why would you allow thoughts that steal your joy to enter and live inside your mind?

How can you become a better you if you're always living in your past? Spending every day regretting every mistake you've ever made is no way to live. We've all said and done things we wish we hadn't; we've hurt people, we've acted selfishly, we've lied and we've all judged others. No one is immune from making mistakes. Admit yours and learn from them, but don't keep beating yourself up about them for the rest of your life – by doing that you're poisoning yourself.

Let it go. The things that have happened in the past and are not happening right now. Let it go. If you want to be free, to find peace, stop locking yourself into the prison of your past. Release the heavy weight from your back. Let it go.

I understand there are people out there who may not let you forget mistakes you have made. If you have those toxic people in your life who make you feel alone, hopeless or strange, then don't waste your energy on them. There's nothing strange about you – what's strange is having to deal with people like that. Don't let those people invade your mind like a virus. It'll only affect the quality of your life in every other area. Show that you are brave enough to let it go: show that you're strong enough to enjoy your life to the full.

Focus on the good. Those who you seem to think are having amazing lives, haven't just got lucky. When one course of action doesn't work for them, they move on quickly and focus on the next positive. Whenever negative thoughts or painful memories surface, take a baseball bat and send them soaring into the sky away from you. Don't cheat on your future with your past; it's over.

Living with guilt doesn't do anything productive. It doesn't help you live better, it only makes you struggle more. Guilt will drain you emotionally and physically; it will wear you out. When you're letting guilt drain you, you won't pursue dreams and goals – you just get stuck. Depression can work overtime in this area. It knows guilt will keep you from your peace. Depression would love nothing more than for you to go through the rest of your life pushing against yourself.

Guilt and shame are far more likely to cause destructive behaviours than cure them. We need to get our heads and hearts around that as a culture. When we mess up, when we've hurt someone, we acknowledge what we've done, we apologize, we learn from it and move on. You can't wallow in something that's already happened. You can't change it.

It's harder to defend yourself when the voice of accusation is stronger on the inside. Guilt isn't just dealing with what others are saying about you, it's about what you are saying about yourself. It's the struggle inside you. Have you ever thought to yourself, *What was I thinking?! What on earth was I doing?*

Guilt is a wasted emotion; don't let it waste your time. You can make amends, of course, and you can do better. But guilt solves nothing. Acknowledgment isn't the same as guilt. Build guilt resilience by replacing the feelings of guilt with acknowledgment.

I know from personal experiences that it can be really easy to forgive other people but a real struggle to forgive ourselves. We'd all love to be able to take back our past mistakes, but would you want to take back all the past lessons you've learnt from those experiences? I imagine not. We want the lessons but not the experiences. Realize there are lessons learned. When you don't judge your past, it's a lot easier to accept what's taken place. The mistakes have happened. Let's change how we respond to them rather than dwell on them.

Guilt is a heavy burden but it can only exist in places where you care.

Know who you are today. Have the self-awareness, the presence to look at yourself honestly and accept you've made mistakes without punishing yourself or spending your time every day in the past, living there in the pain of what you've got wrong.

There are only two things under our control and they're our thoughts and actions in the present moment. Everything else is out of our hands: what people think of us, how people behave and also the past. We can't go back and change things – believe me, I've looked into it! As much as *Back to the Future* is one of my favourite movies of all time, time travelling to correct our mistakes is not currently on the table. We need to let it go.

When you don't forgive yourself, you are helping depression do its job.

If you want to create something new, don't spend your time and energy trying to tear down the old. Use that energy and time to build the new. Use that energy and time in building you.

CHAPTER 9

After being attacked, it took me a few months to recover. It had actually knocked my confidence to go out socially during that time so I hadn't been drinking for a while. Cheaper than rehab, I suppose!

During that break from alcohol, I was wanting to learn more about this Jesus guy (spoiler alert: he dies and comes back from the dead).

Even as I looked more into Christianity, I had doubts and felt like I could be wasting my time. How could I ever believe in things like Noah's Ark and be taken seriously? I remember thinking to myself, *How would you get all those animals on the same boat? I can't even get my dog in the shower.* But there was something in me that just wouldn't give up learning more about Christianity and who Jesus was.

All I knew for sure was that I had experienced a surreal, overwhelming sense of peace. It felt amazing. I had never had a high like it before and I needed more of it.

After the attack I had suffered, I was also feeling incredibly anxious as well as dealing with this lingering depression. I hadn't had any medication for a while and I knew I needed to get back on it – and not mix the medication with alcohol if I really wanted to get better. I had made the decision myself to stop seeing Dr Galt when I was feeling slightly better. My naïve mind told me I didn't need her help anymore. I was better and was able to go out and enjoy myself again. I cancelled my appointments with her, ignored her phone calls and stopped the medication she was giving me cold turkey (which is a really big mistake). So it is hardly surprisingly that I felt pretty bad at going back to see her – like a dog with its tail between its legs. I was in the waiting room with a feeling that I can only describe as reminiscent of sitting outside the head teacher's office at school, knowing you'd done something wrong.

I thought it would be awkward seeing her under the circumstances but it didn't feel like that at all. Dr Galt once again welcomed me with open arms. She's a brilliant doctor. I knew I could trust her. I was able to open up about coming close to hanging myself and told her about the attack. I was put back on medication; that was a relief. She pleaded with me not to drink any alcohol whilst I was going through this. I promised her I wouldn't. I felt like I was getting a second chance to not mess things up by binge drinking this time.

But I was less thrilled with what Dr Galt mentioned next. She said, "I feel like it's essential you have a supportive network around you, with people you would feel comfortable talking to. I'm going to book you in at the Elm Centre."

CHAPTER 10

It's a strange time that we're living in right now. People in the countries that have the most, feel like they have the least. People that live in countries that have the most reasons to be happy, seem to experience the least happiness. I believe this is due to comparison. Whether it be because of social media, money or our own personal pride, we can be guilty of comparing ourselves to everyone who has more.

Comparison is the thief of joy.

Never compare yourself to others. It doesn't matter how great you feel you are, if you are not grateful for who you are and what you have, then you'll never be happy. There's always going to be someone who has more money than you; there will always be someone who has more followers than you, someone fitter than you, better looking than you. If you are always comparing yourself, you'll lose every time. Run your own race and be happy for all others to run theirs, in their own time and in their own way. Happy people don't have the best of everything, they make the best of everything.

One thing other people will *never* have over you: they are not you! Your greatest asset is that you're unique. And when you are free to be exactly as you are, that's the greatest way to live.

Appreciation and gratitude are a great relief from depression or any low states. Depression does not sit well with gratitude; I know which one I choose.

Don't set yourself rules about being happy. If you say, "I can only be happy if X, Y and Z happen in my life," you're setting yourself up for failure and unhappiness because life will always throw challenges and obstacles your way.

Social media worries me, especially the effect it may be having on the younger generation, and I worry that the use of filters isn't healthy at all. If filters can make you look like a supermodel in one swipe, I worry it will lead to people filtering things in their own lives, like exaggerating everything to make themselves seem bigger and better and leaving out all the things they are struggling with and causing them pain.

The most destructive problem I feel depression can ever give someone, more so than any of the cardinal sins in my opinion, is self-pity. I believe that self-pity is the worst possible emotion that anyone can have and the most destructive. Self-pity will destroy relationships, motivation and anything that's good, leaving only itself. It's very easy to feel sorry for ourselves, we've all been hard done by and have instances where things are unfair and where we feel underappreciated. They may well be true, but to pity yourself over these things is doing yourself enormous disservice. It's incredibly self-destructive.

If you have experienced pain, it will generate energy that you can use against yourself – or for yourself.

CHAPTER 11

The more we can talk shamelessly and openly about depression and mental health, the better. I was someone who for years hadn't told anyone close to me just how much I was struggling. It was hard enough to tell Dr Galt and my best friend but that was it. The staff at the school that I worked at made me feel as though it was something that I really couldn't share openly, as it wasn't normal and was something people wouldn't understand.

It's important to be open about mental health, as it can trigger life-changing conversations. You'll be surprised how many people can relate to the topic, as almost everyone has some kind of direct experience of a mental health problem. It might not be their own but someone in their family, someone in their circle of friends may have been someone who has gone through it.

It seems to be a lot harder for men to talk about mental health, and it seems that this is why suicide rates among men are a lot higher than they are among women. Suicide is the greatest cause of death in men under 40 in the UK – greater than cancer, greater than any type of heart or lung disease, greater than car accidents or anything else. That's a really serious issue. We still live in a culture where men aren't encouraged to be vulnerable. We joke about man flu and talk about manning up, we're led to believe that men need to be tough – the strong and silent gender – and that they don't have deep and complex feelings. Although some would say there are a lot of social and economic advantages to being a male, I believe there is an emotional handicap. We do have deep feelings but we just don't always express them. Unfortunately, suicide is just the tip of an enormous, ugly iceberg. Underneath the surface is the real bulk of this floating monster, which comprises all the things that lead to suicide. We need to change attitudes and admit to what we are really feeling so that we can deal with mental health issues with care, understanding and inner strength.

Men are three times more likely to commit suicide than women. If you feel you don't have anyone you can speak to, then you're more likely to resort to what can feel like the only other option.

I saw a video recently on YouTube of Dwayne "The Rock" Johnson, the movie actor and professional wrestler, talking about his struggles with depression. It was a really big eye opener for me to see this giant of a man being able to share his feelings so openly. For men out there struggling, this is an object lesson. This guy is handsome, stacked, rich, popular – it would be hard to find a more "manly" guy, and yet he can admit he finds aspects of life difficult. We need to encourage men to realize that it's not embarrassing to be experiencing these types of feelings and it doesn't make them "not manly enough".

There doesn't need to be an absence of hope.

CHAPTER 12

It was my first day at the Elm Centre and I felt completely out of place. I was in a group therapy session with about eight other patients. I felt very awkward about being in a group with these people. I was at school before everything got politically correct, and in certain classes we would have what was known as the "thick table" – what a ghastly expression! Of course, it was nothing to do with the table; it was where the so-called "intellectually challenged" pupils would all sit together. Obviously, that would never happen in schools now, and rightly so.

If anyone was ever a bit cheeky in class, or not listening to the teacher, that's where we'd be sent. I can remember on many occasions pleading with my teachers, "Please sir, don't put me on the thick table!"

As bad as it sounds, as I looked around the patients in this group therapy session, it reminded me of that table. I was clearly with vulnerable people. There was one girl who kept rocking back and forth on her chair and wouldn't make eye contact with anyone. I had only to come into the Elm for certain sessions during the day but quite a few of the others were full-time residents at the centre. I felt very uncomfortable. I felt we all had very separate issues and couldn't see how this would help with my depression at all.

There was another guy called Stewart who must have been in his late 40s. He seemed perhaps the most vulnerable in the group. He was clinging onto a teddy bear that he called Ben, named him after Michael Jackson's song "Ben" about a pet rat. Stewart also had an old-looking blanket in his other hand. There was another girl with a shaved head – I kept catching her eye. I tried to be subtle but I couldn't help but look at the numerous cuts all along her arms. She was clearly someone who was self-harming.

Most of the patients in the group were looking at me, probably because I was a new face. I began to think to myself, *I shouldn't be here. Yes, I know I'm depressed but I feel like I'm with a bunch of people who clearly can't look after themselves.*

There was one friendly face smiling at me. She looked familiar. Then it dawned on me just who it was. Her name was Claire, and we had studied theatre together a few years earlier. We didn't know each other well, but the first thing I noticed was how skinny she had become. She had always been slim but she looked like a skeleton and unbelievably fragile.

The group sessions started. I was briefly introduced by one of the counsellors there before things opened up with a guy called Loie. I'd say Loie was probably in his late 30s and had schizophrenia. Loie spoke about how he believed the American foreign intelligence service, the CIA, was planning to kill him. He was a huge conspiracy theorist; he spoke about how the US government was behind the assassination of former president John F Kennedy, the 9/11 attacks and many celebrity deaths. He felt because he knew "the truth" about what was happening that the CIA were planning to silence him.

Loie could never be left alone as he would be in extreme panic. He wouldn't even use the toilet – he felt that would be the perfect opportunity for the CIA to strike. He hadn't used the toilet in months; he had to wear adult incontinence pants.

Next to speak was a man called Paul. Paul was actually a 60-year-old Church of England vicar. His dependence on alcohol was affecting his life and his job. He opened up about this in the session.

"The thing is, the parishioners were all complaining that the communion wine was going missing. One old lady said there was a hobo sleeping in the church graveyard. I had to pretend to go and look for him but it was me!"

Claire was speaking next. I listened keenly. I wondered what had happened to her since college. As she spoke, it appeared that her battle had pre-dated college and she'd had issues with her mental health since secondary school. I didn't go to Claire's school, but she spoke about how she used to get teased about being fat and had struggled with her weight and food for years. Her battle was anorexia.

She opened up about how horribly she was bullied. I remember it made me feel very angry and I think it was the first time I really realized the effect bullying can have on someone. I certainly wasn't a bully at school but can remember on different occasions being a part of mean pranks on people and laughing at those who were getting picked on, blissfully unaware of the effect it may be having. I hated to see the effect bullying had on Claire. I could feel the pain in her voice.

When it got to my turn to speak in the group, I didn't say much.

"I've just been feeling really down over the last year or so," I said and didn't feel like sharing much more than that, despite being pushed a few times by the counsellor who was leading the session. I think she soon realized I wasn't going to say much else and moved on.

After the group session concluded, we were put in pairs to talk more to each other and encouraged to share more about our experiences. I remember hoping to be paired with Claire. I felt it would be a lot less awkward with her and we would probably be able to have a productive conversation.

"Lawrence, let's put you with Loie," one of the nurses said.

"For fuck sake," I muttered to myself.

CHAPTER 13

This probably sounds a bit cheesy, but I really think as a species we need to collectively emphasize and re-evaluate what it means to be kinder to each other. I mean, nobody teaches you that, it's rare. Yes, you might get taught at school to be nice, learn lessons at a church, and working in an office means adhering to certain standards of behaviour.

But I just feel in society today there's not that emphasis on kindness and just being friendly. When you're nice to someone or someone is nice to you, it's always a good feeling. Whether it involves holding the door open for someone or helping someone get down some stairs with a baby in a pram – you get a good feeling from helping someone and it's so easy to do. It doesn't cost anything and I feel it is so underrated.

Admittedly, recently I was on the underground and I looked at a guy sitting opposite me as I got on and simply said, "All right, mate," but he just stared at me. To be honest, initially I was angry; immediately I was thinking, *What a prick*. But you've just got to let it go and feel sorry for miserable buggers like that.

We all want to feel good, and from helping people and being kind, we can achieve that. It not only makes whoever you're kind to feel good but it also makes you feel amazing as well. It instantly makes you feel good about yourself no matter how you're currently feeling.

There have been moments in my life where I've felt terrible, where I've made huge mistakes, fucked up, failed or just felt lost and like absolute crap. When you're feeling like that it's worth asking yourself what's preventing you from feeling good in that moment. Sometimes we don't allow ourselves to move on from fucking up as we feel we need to learn from it. Some people can allow themselves to wallow in those feelings for their lifetime. Why, on the other side of that, can we not remind ourselves of the good deeds we have done too?

There's nothing wrong with telling yourself:

"You know what, I feel great because I helped that old lady out with her shopping today."

Being kind doesn't have to diminish competition. You can be up for a part against someone or interviewing for the same job but still show kindness to that person. There doesn't need to be so much bitchiness, jealousy and unpleasantness in working hard to achieve something.

You don't have to be a dick to get things done.

CHAPTER 14

Once you have experienced depression, there is always the possibility that it will rear its ugly head uninvited. Whenever it decides to make an appearance, you'll feel empty and life will just feel like it's slowing down. It can surprise you with a visit for no reason.

When the rest of the world seems to be enjoying life in colour, it feels as though you can only see it in black and white. Activities that usually bring you pleasure suddenly cease to be enjoyable. Depression can chew up your appetite, memory and ability to concentrate. With depression holding you down, it feels like doing anything or going anywhere requires superhuman strength. At those times, I'd have to take naps in the day because I was so exhausted and couldn't figure out why.

In social occasions, depression would sniff out what confidence I had and tear it away. This is why I felt like I had to drink to be social. No one would want quiet, boring, miserable Lawrence to hang out with. Alcohol gave me a short-term buzz, but the comedown from that wasn't worth it and the depression came back tenfold.

Covering up your depression so people don't find out requires far too much energy. Keeping up an emotional lie is exhausting. It can make you irritable and difficult to be around. It'll wake you up with repetitive, negative thinking whilst reminding you how exhausted you will be the next day.

Depression is not about feeling a bit down, sad or blue; at its worst it's about being devoid of any sense of feeling altogether.

Don't let your dark cloud get bigger.

CHAPTER 15

"So, you really think if you go to the toilet the CIA will assassinate you?" I asked Loie, certainly a question I never saw myself asking in my lifetime.

"It's inevitable," he replied quickly. "They just need the most convenient opportunity."

"Wouldn't that be when you sleep?" I questioned.

"I don't sleep at night. I sleep about four hours in the day. Even the CIA wouldn't assassinate me in broad daylight."

I remember trying several different techniques to try and encourage him to the toilet.

"What if I guarded the toilet? What if I peed in the urinal next to you? What if we communicated on walkie talkies while you peed?

These were all ideas I suggested, but to Loie they were all far too risky. Not only for his safety, but for mine, so he felt.

As I tried my hardest to make a breakthrough with Loie, it just seemed hopeless. But then I had my own eureka moment – well, that sounds like it was a plan, but actually I had absolutely no idea whether it would work or not. It also may well have got me into trouble. But I wasn't too fussed – I really didn't want to be there anyway, so it was certainly worth a try. I had a quick glance around me to make sure no one was listening in on our conversation. I decided to enter Loie's very real reality.

"Look Loie. I'm going to be honest with you. I'm going to tell you something now that is classified information. You need to promise this stays completely between us. It's a matter of national security. Do you understand?"

Loie leant in keenly towards me. "Absolutely," he whispered back.

"Loie, I'm agent P – I work with MI6," I stated, glancing back over my shoulder. "I'm here undercover."

"I knew it," Loie responded.

"Really?" I asked with surprise, as it was something I had made up in my head about 30 seconds previously, but I quickly slipped back into character and fortunately he didn't notice.

"I knew you looked federal," he answered.

"I see, well, we have been watching the CIA monitoring you very carefully. We are aware of it. You're right to be cautious. But I've been sent in here to tell you that you're currently absolutely safe and protected here," I continued to whisper.

"I am?" Loie responded. His voice cracked, you could clearly tell knowing he was safe was an emotional assurance for him, either that or just the thought of someone else finally believing his fears.

"You're under MI6 protection, Loie. Relationships between us and the United States are good. They aren't going to jeopardize that by killing you. I'm here to pass that message on to you. I assure you, Loie, it's completely safe for you to sleep at night and completely safe for you to use the toilet. I think you should even try and go now, with the assurance that I'm here to protect you."

"No, it's too risky," Loie replied nervously.

"Trust me, Loie, now is the perfect moment. I'll check the room is clear, then on my signal you have to go for it. Understood?" I insisted.

I didn't give Loie a chance to say much back to me at that point. I stood up and made my way to the communal toilet, trying to act as "James Bond" as I possibly could. To be completely honest, I was even starting to get into character of my MI6 persona. I slowly opened the toilet door, peeking in and out as I did so. I remember one of the nurses looking at me oddly.

"Just checking no one's in here," I smiled at her. I didn't want to be too over the top, otherwise they'd probably lock me in as a full-time resident too.

Having checked the toilet, I gave Loie our pre-arranged signal, which to my memory was a closed fist to my chest followed by a point towards him.

"LET'S DO THIS!" Loie screamed as he ran towards me.

Well there goes my plan to do this as quietly, subtly and as unsuspicious as possible, I thought to myself. *I may as well fully invest in this role now.*

"GO! GO! GO!" I called back as Loie rushed past me and slammed the toilet door, locking it behind him.

I smiled and chuckled to myself as I leant against the wall. I never thought I'd be so satisfied to hear another man urinate.

CHAPTER 16

I write this on Friday the 17 July 2020. Today I've woken up feeling pretty crap. I thought it might be useful to include this in my writing to show that, although I'm in a much better place with my mental health, I can still get these very dark, bad days where depression has slowly wandered in like a thief in the night.

As I feel absolute pants right now, I will try a few techniques that usually work for me. They help me get on with my day rather than spending hours looking at my bedroom ceiling, replaying every regret I have in my life over and over again in my mind.

I remind myself that today is just a bad day for it. The weather inside my head is just really rubbish. I remind myself that I've seen much worse, much darker and much more hopeless days. As I write this now in my bed, I find that this in itself is already helping me – just letting my feelings spill out with good old pen and paper. I suppose it's a lot cheaper than therapy.

When I put this pen down and close my notepad, I will spend some time praying and meditating, asking for peace to come into my body like a waterfall and flush away these depressive feelings. I will get up, make a healthy breakfast and, although it's the last thing I feel like doing right now, I will go for a long run.

I feel as though if you're going to do one thing to vastly improve any mental health struggles you're going through, then that is to exercise. By physically moving, your physiology changes and with that so does your brain. Get outside and exercise every single day. Your body needs it, your brain needs it and your mental health needs it.

Get outside, get your heart rate up, breathe, and get out of your house, which may be causing some issues with your depression. Doing that every day is vital. You don't even have to run: go to the gym or take an aerobics class. Get outside and walk your dog, walk with your friend for a couple of miles. Doing that every single day is healthy for your mind, changes your physical environment, and also creates routine and momentum in your life. Like I say, I know when you're at your worst with depression, exercise is the last thing you want to do – believe me, I get it. But I can't stress enough the importance of it to give you a brighter tomorrow.

Anyway, wish me luck. Here's to a brighter tomorrow.

CHAPTER 17

"Get the fuck off me!" was echoing in the centre as I arrived the next morning. I walked past one of the meeting rooms to head into the communal room. I saw a man being restrained by four different nurses. It was hard to say for sure how old he was. I would have guessed mid-30s perhaps, but he looked so troubled, tired and worn out that he could have well been younger. His eyes were bloodshot and I remember feeling that his eyes showed what a tortured soul he was.

Stewart came out of the communal room clutching Ben, his bear, to observe what the noise was. He was starting to panic and began to cry hysterically like a small child. He curled up his bear right up next to his face, seemingly for reassurance, protection or comfort.

The nurses looked like they were struggling to restrain this guy. "Is everything okay?" I asked, wondering if I could help in any way. The guy's violent-looking eyes targeted me and he started aiming his aggression my way.

"Who the fuck are you? You good-doer prick. What the fuck are you looking at?" he yelled at me.

One of the nurses looked at me and, in a fluster, said, "Shut that door now." As she said this, I saw one of the other nurses preparing a shot of some kind, seemingly to try and calm him down or sedate him. As I went to shut the door, one of the other nurses rushed towards us and shut the door behind her.

"It's probably best you head to the common room, if that's okay," said the nurse.

"Who was that?" I asked.

"Ah, yes, you wouldn't have met Ian yet," she sighed.

"What's wrong with him?" I added.

"That's not for here," she bluntly replied before once again ushering me and Stewart, who was still crying hysterically, towards the common room.

"Come on then, Stewart," I said as I started to walk towards the common room. Stewart held out his hand – he clearly wanted me to hold it and escort him there. *What the fuck have I got myself into*, I thought as I reluctantly held Stewart's hand and led him to the common room.

As soon as we were inside, I was in for another unpleasant surprise. I saw Loie sitting watching television. I put my free hand up to acknowledge him, but couldn't help but feel he looked at me nervously, trying to avoid making eye contact with me. I knew he had seen me, yet for whatever reason he was pretending he hadn't. It soon occurred to me that Loie had told someone my little MI6 story and was feeling guilty. The centre's manager walked into the communal room.

"Good morning, Lawrence. Could I have a word, please?"

CHAPTER 18

Treat depression as if it were a person. When I started to view depression as a person, I felt it helped me tremendously. When you realize you're dealing with a person that's not yourself, you're on your way to beating it. Depression's objective is to torment and torture you, to isolate you, to keep you from finding hope and peace. Depression is a liar. Separate what is you and what is depression.

By killing yourself, you're never killing depression, depression is killing you. It completes its objective.

The characteristics of depression are to entice, harass, torment, compel, enslave, defile, deceive and to push you to a breaking point.

Depression will be really possessive of you. It doesn't want you to see your friends and family; it wants you to be completely influenced by it in isolation. If you allow depression to bog you down with loneliness on top of everything else, you will find yourself in a world of appalling pain. Do not let it cut you off.

CHAPTER 19

I spoke earlier about being ashamed of being a sensitive kid. But as I've grown up, I truly believe that if you're a sensitive person you should embrace that. Sensitive souls have great empathy. We feel the sadness of our loved ones when they're going through a hard time. Again, it's tougher for men to be labelled as sensitive; as guys we are supposed to be aggressive and competitive. Sadly, the notion that a man can be both sensitive and strong is an alien concept. As someone who considers himself sensitive, I feel we make up a group of people who process the world in a vivid way.

Sensitivity shouldn't be seen as a weakness. Telling people they're too sensitive achieves nothing. It's like going up to someone who's bald and saying, "Mate, you're bald." They're still going to be bald after you've said this. It changes nothing. Sensitivity is not a flaw, it's not an unfortunate Achilles' heel. Where would we be without such sensitive souls such as Martin Luther King Jr, Mahatma Gandhi and Albert Einstein? Without their beautiful empathy I imagine the world would be a slightly darker shade. By trying to hide my sensitivity when I was younger, purely to fit in, I was miserable.

I think as a society we need to embrace sensitivity, not to label sensitives as "snowflakes". Let's come together to rewrite the negative cultural narrative of sensitivity and turn it into a positive one. Erase the notion that it is a weakness, acknowledge its many strengths. We should all be able to embrace our softer sides. If, like me, you've ever felt you're too sensitive, stop. Stop trying to toughen up, stop hiding and don't feel weird. There's nothing weird about you; it's not you that should be considered wrong. Step up and share your loving, sensitive side with the world. We need more sensitive souls to pave a way through the troubled times ahead. The world needs to be a gentler one.

CHAPTER 20

"So, last night Loie told me, along with some of the other members of staff and patients, that he was under MI6 protection. Would you care to explain this?" the centre leader asked me in her office. For a moment, I wasn't sure whether to come clean or play dumb. I thought that maybe I could just pretend to have no idea what she was on about, but I thought that may come back on Loie and go against his mental health progression at the centre if they thought he was plucking out wild lies from thin air. So, I decided to try and justify my behaviour.

"I mean, I thought it might help him with going to the toilet and stuff," I explained. "At the end of the day, he was able to go to the toilet and he hasn't been able to, right? So, there's no harm done."

"The problem is, Lawrence, by playing along with Loie's delusions, you're very much adding to the problem. We are trying to get him to process reality. What's real and what's not. By fuelling these wild theories of his you're taking away all the hard work the staff have been doing with him. Do you understand?"

"I appreciate what you're saying. But he's able to use the toilet now, right? Maybe it was the case of trying something different with him? He's still clearly got the belief that the American intelligence are trying to kill him, so I thought that perhaps entering his world might help," I explained.

"But it doesn't help, Lawrence, and can I please remind you that you're not a member of staff here or qualified to make such an assumption. You're here as a patient," she went on.

"Look, to be honest with you, I don't even want to be here," I said bluntly.

"But yet you're here of your own accord? So, you must be wanting the help we provide to make you better?"

"Not really. I kind of felt I owed my doctor to give this a go," I sighed.

"I think this is helping you a lot more than you believe it is. You have been shutting yourself off and hiding this pain all to yourself. Now you have people around you, a support network," she said.

"I feel like I'm being sent to the fucking headteacher's office because I've been naughty. I was just trying to help the guy out," I said. I was starting to get more frustrated.

"Lawrence, it's not like that at all. But it's my duty to explain to you the damage your actions can potentially cause to someone as vulnerable as Loie."

When that was said to me, I blew a bit of a gasket. I'm quite a calm person usually, especially when sober. But the fact it was insinuated I could be causing Loie "damage" – I was really pissed off. I'm not particularly proud of how I acted next.

"Well, fuck this then. I'm going," I said as I stood up from my chair.

"Lawrence, please stay here and calm down. We are planning some important sessions for you today."

"I don't want your sessions. This whole thing has been a complete waste of time. I've done my bit. I've given this a go. You've put me in a group full of nutters and the whole thing here is a circus," I said as I headed for the door. "I'm leaving. I'm allowed to any time I want. I'm not one of your fucking residents here."

"Lawrence, I must inform you that if you leave, I will be informing your GP and I will be writing on your case file AMA, that you're leaving against medical advice."

"And I'll be writing IDGAFF. I don't give a flying fuck," I retorted as I slammed her office door as I left.

I headed straight for the door of the centre, ready to just walk out on the whole thing. Claire was in the common room as I walked out.

"Is everything okay?" she asked, but I blanked her and continued to head towards the door.

As I got closer to the door, the man who I saw being restrained by the nurses on my arrival was walking down the corridor by the meeting room.

"Sorry about earlier, mate. It's just one of those days," he said. I just continued past him, not responding at all, and went to open the door.

"Can you release the door for me, please?" I said with gritted teeth to one of the nurses by the door.

"Oh, are you done for the day?" she asked, puzzled.

"Oh, I'm done all right," I answered.

The centre's manager was walking up the corridor behind me. "Lawrence, I think you should stay. Calm down, get yourself a drink and we'll talk about this in a little while," she said calmly.

"No, thank you. Please open the door," I requested.

"Lawrence, I really think that …"

"OPEN THE FUCKING DOOR!" I screamed.

I was feeling a rising panic. Yesterday I was able to walk in and out relatively freely because I had self-admitted to the centre. Now I felt like a prisoner. I wasn't able to walk out and I was now being instructed to stay.

"YOU CAN'T KEEP ME HERE!" I continued to shout as I kicked the door. I was growing frustrated as more nurses seemed to rush to the scene in an attempt to calm me down. But that only made my panic grow worse. *These fuckers are going to try and keep me here full-time*, I thought to myself.

I darted back to the common room. There must have been about five members of staff behind me, trying to keep me from leaving. As I marched into the common room, I headed towards the communal garden. Loie seemed in a bit of a panic when he saw what was going on.

"Oh no, I've blown his cover! I'm so sorry!" I heard him cry as I opened the door to the garden.

"Lawrence? Do you need to talk?" I heard Claire say as I walked past her. I looked at the garden wall and slowly ran towards it, hopping over it and heading up a little alley that led into the town, which I took and headed home.

I never did return to the Elm Centre. Obviously now, looking back, I wish I had handled the situation better. I have no doubt that all the staff there had my best interests at heart and wanted to help me. Anyone who really knows me, knows I'm a relatively calm guy. But in that moment, I was overwhelmed by all the emotions I was going through. The intense depression, the anxiety, the fear and the panic. At that moment, it all got too much for me. I just had to run.

CHAPTER 21

It's not easy being depressed. It's not easy loving someone who is depressed either. Sometimes being there for them and doing things for them that you think might be helpful actually aren't. The intentions are good, it's no one's fault, but I think there are some important things to know about loving someone who is depressed. There are things you can do that are helpful, but also things to be aware of that may not be helpful. At the same time, it's really hard for you to know what your loved one is experiencing.

There are a few things I would advise avoiding saying to a depressed loved one:

"You just need to get out of the house."

"Think positive."

"Get some fresh air, you'll feel better."

Saying things like this won't make your loved one feel better. Always bear in mind that depression isn't just a matter of having a bad day or feeling sad. It is a mental illness that is completely overwhelming. It's nothing you can just walk off. Saying things like this to someone who's depressed can actually make them feel more helpless because they know they can't just get over it but feel perhaps they should.

Some things that are helpful to say are simply:

"I love you."

"I care for you."

"I believe in you."

"I'm here for you."

"You are strong."

"I know you can get through this."

Being honest and genuine in those words of encouragement are really important for someone with depression to hear.

In some ways, it is just human nature to try to offer advice – please resist the temptation. A lot of people like to give advice, not so many to take it. Even if your words are coming from a good place, these kind of comments are not helpful:

"Eat different food."

"Go see a therapist."

"Have you tried this medication?"

Again, although all these things can really be helpful with treating depression, a loved one telling you what you should do or shouldn't do isn't what you need. Like anyone that tells us what we should or shouldn't be doing, it doesn't feel good, even if it is coming from a good place. It can leave the person feeling helpless and frustrated.

Although things like eating healthy, seeing a doctor and exercise are really important in the fight against depression, instead of saying "you should do this" or "you shouldn't do that", try saying things like:

"Hey, what have you tried?"

"What have you learned about what you're feeling?"

"Have you tried any of these options?"

"I've read that exercising might be helpful, are you interested in hearing more about that? I could send some things over for you to read."

If they say no, then you know without frustrating them too much. Or they might be more positive about this approach and use the opportunity to talk to you on a deeper level about what they're going through without them feeling like they've been told what to and what not to do.

Sometimes, people who are depressed feel like they have to push their loved ones away. I just want to make it as clear as I can that this is not because they don't love you. It's because they're feeling overwhelmed, and it's also because they feel like they don't want to overwhelm you. They feel they don't want to keep putting their crap on you. When going through depression, you feel awful a lot of the time and the last thing you want to do is bring that sadness and those depressive feelings onto your loved ones. They might seemingly disappear for a while, not messaging you, not answering calls, not going out or wanting to see anyone, but again this is not because they care less about you or don't love you – it's because they do. They don't want to be a burden to anyone and they feel bad about it. So typically, when they're going through a particularly bad time with depression, they feel it best to have some space. It's almost like hibernating from the weather in your head.

Again, the best thing to do is just to remind that person how much they're loved, how much you care for them. If they need some space that's fine, but let them know you're available if they need you and let them know you're there to talk when they're ready. Remind them that you're there to support them, because depression will tell them that people don't care about them. It will tell them that people are going to give up on them, people are going to leave them. Those are the lies they will constantly be hearing. So please keep reaffirming your love and support for them.

Loving someone who is depressed can be challenging, upsetting and draining. So, you also need to be taking care of yourself. You need to be able to tell your loved one how you can and can't support them. You don't need to feel it's your job or your responsibility to fix them, because you can't. You're a supporter, not a fixer. It's very different and it's less exhausting because being a supporter is do-able. Thinking you have to change someone and trying to change them doesn't work. You will wear yourself out for nothing. So just being able to tell your loved ones how you can and can't support them is setting up boundaries that work for both of you.

From my own experiences, I can say when I've been going through bad battles with depression, I can cancel plans, leave an event early or pull out of different commitments. When your loved one with depression does that, it can feel really hurtful. You may think, *Oh, they don't care about me, they're not having a good time*, whatever. But just so you know, they are not leaving because they don't like you or they're bored of your company. They're leaving because the depression has come over them, and it's made them feel like they just have to be alone. They feel like they can't be in a certain environment or situation.

If they cancel plans at the last minute, it's just that they can't muster up the energy to go out and be sociable, to have to put on an act. I can't emphasize enough how exhausting that is. Know that it not personal.

I know it can be really hard, especially if it happens regularly. But just try and be able to say, "Okay, you know what, I know you're dealing with something right now. I'm here for you, I love and support you. Is there anything I can do? How can I help?" Those words go *so* far. They are so meaningful.

Never blame yourself. You cannot be blamed for someone else's depression. You can't make someone depressed. It's a depressive disorder, you can't cause it. You can't blame yourselves and feel responsible. Feeling like that will cause you so much stress and anxiety as you're trying to support a loved one. So, know that if you have a loved one who is depressed, that's all. It's not your fault.

CHAPTER 22

A few days after leaving the centre, I had agreed to meet Claire in a nearby park while she had a lunch break. She had been messaging me to check in and see that I was okay. I arrived at the park, seeing her sitting with a bottle of water on the park bench. At this stage, I still felt I had made the right decision by quitting the treatment I was getting.

"How are you feeling?" Claire asked me.

"Surviving," I smiled. "Guess I caused quite the commotion, eh?"

"I wouldn't worry about it too much. It's not like it's completely out of the ordinary there anyway," she answered back.

"Is Loie all right?" I was surprised I even asked that question, I didn't realize I could genuinely worry about how Loie was doing.

"I mean, he wants to sleep with a gun under his pillow. But other than that, he's coping fine. Maybe you can sort him out with a special gadget eh, Mr Bond?" she joked.

"I thought it might help him," I sighed.

"I know you did," Claire smiled back.

"How are you doing anyway? Do you find the people there helpful?" I asked Claire.

"Yes, but sometimes the patients are just as helpful. You should know that with Loie. Didn't it take your mind off the way you were feeling? Even if just for a little while?" she asked.

She was completely right: by focusing on Loie for that short amount of time, I was completely zoned out from my own depressive feelings. I was purely thinking of how I might be able to help him.

"I suppose you're right, actually," I smiled.

"It's nice to have those moments where you just slip away from it and forget," she sighed.

"Are you getting better?" I asked her.

"Not really, but it's nice to have people around me. I'm sleep-deprived, stressed and just want to rest," she answered. "But it's important to talk, Lawrence. Sometimes in the past I have felt like I've asked for help and been ignored. At secondary school I was bullied and by college my mental health was really struggling: self-harming, trying to take my life. I felt I needed to do something. I needed to be around people who would make things positive again, away from the people who made me feel awful."

"You shouldn't listen to people like that, Claire," I remember saying. "The people that bullied you are not worth a second thought," I added.

"I always believed them, though, I always thought I was fat and hideous."

I'm not sure why, but at this point I decided to kiss Claire. It was a kiss like I hadn't experienced before. It was gentle, unseedy and was an expression of genuinely caring for someone. It lasted just a few seconds.

"I'm sorry, I'm not exactly sure why I did that," I said as I backed away. I was worried I might have overwhelmed her. I remember being conscious again that I wasn't considering someone else's feelings – something I felt like I struggled with.

"Don't be sorry," she smiled, "I'm not complaining."

Claire went on to tell me something that gives me goosebumps thinking about to this day.

"You know Loz, I remember being jealous of the butterflies. I envied them. I envied how they could just hide away and change their appearance. Doesn't matter how they felt or what they were before, they could always just hide away and turn into these beautiful things that could fly away and be free." A tear started to run down her face. "I hate feeling like this so much, Lawrence. It's a life that I wouldn't wish on anyone else." I embraced Claire with a hug as she gently began to sob.

"You're stronger than you think Claire. This world needs more people like you in it," I said to her.

"What? Another weirdo?" she joked through her tears.

"Absolutely," I smiled, "Aren't most of the greatest people in history pretty nuts? We all have a flicker of weirdness. Maybe we should embrace it rather than trying to hide it. Hiding our weird little quirks makes us just like everybody else, and that sounds rather pants to me."

That was the last time I ever saw Claire. She went on struggling with her mental health and moved to Wales. She was sectioned for a while due to concerns about how serious her anorexia had become. She was very brave. She spoke out about her battles; she wrote for the Huffington Post and had her words published by Penguin. Although we never saw each other again, we continued to message each other on and off. We were both getting involved in writing. She was writing about mental health and I was writing children's stories; we shared our writing and gave each other feedback. I believe Claire was sent to a specialized ward in Coventry as her mental health started to deteriorate. In her last messages to me, she told me she was struggling being so far away from home and she was feeling very unwell.

For the next few months, I reached out to Claire several times. I wasn't getting a response and was becoming increasingly worried about her, but trusted she was in the right place, getting the right care. I missed talking to her. She was the friend I could talk to about anything and know I'd be completely unjudged. We spoke about our struggles together; I could talk to her about Disney and reading and writing. Sadly, I never was able to have those conversations again.

It was not long before I got the news that I dreaded. Claire had lost her battle with her mental health and was no longer with us. It was heartbreaking news. Claire Greaves was a brave, beautiful and kind soul. She was almost too good for this world. She cared about people, she was passionate about changing the stigma attached to mental health, especially eating disorders. Claire wrote articles that I urge you to read, and made public appearances, speaking out about her own demons in the hope she could make a difference and help people, to make people aware that they weren't alone. I urge you all to go onto Youtube and search "Claire Greaves" to watch some of her inspiring talks on the topic that took her life.

A few days after receiving the sad news about Claire, I returned to the bench where we'd sat together a few years earlier. I sat and thought about her. Could I have tried harder to reach her with my messages? Could I have gone to visit her? But sadly, I know that there's nothing I could have done to have saved Claire; I don't think there's anything anyone could have done. Her mental illness had dragged her to a level where she just couldn't cope anymore.

I sat on the bench and questioned everything again. If God was real, why would he let someone as precious as Claire, who had so much more to give, battle with so many demons in her life to the point where she just couldn't cope? What was the point? They say the good die young, but where's the justice in that? I remember sitting on that bench, thinking, *I'm going to go out and get absolutely hammered tonight.*

Just as I was thinking that, I looked at the arm of the bench and my heart skipped a beat. There, perching next to me, was the most beautiful butterfly. A tear ran down my face, but it was a happy tear. I even recall laughing. I must have looked a right nutter. The butterfly started to hover as I looked at it. I put out my hand and it landed on my finger for a few seconds before fluttering away. In that moment, I knew Claire was at peace and she was free. I stood up laughing as I watched the butterfly soar into the sky. I like to think Claire was looking down at me, laughing too.

Now whenever I see a butterfly, I think of the beautiful Claire Greaves. Fly high, angel. 1992–2018.

CHAPTER 23

I was more invested than ever in learning about Christianity after Claire's death. I just couldn't fathom that we are on the earth purely by accident. The more I thought about the earth, the more I believed that there must be more to it and kept coming back to the experience I had when I was attacked and what that was.

I started by learning more about Jesus and his teachings. I started trying out churches. It took me a while to find one where I felt settled. Some churches I tried out were a bit too big for my liking and almost felt like a student gig environment, with lots of music and sets from different performers. I'm sure this works for some people, it just didn't for me. I'm from a performing arts world as it is, I didn't want to connect that into a new church life for me as well. I went to one church where I felt the people were very judgemental, and that wasn't right for me either. I almost felt like the guys my age in attendance didn't like the fact I was in my late 20s, coming into church hungover, wearing shades and wanting to learn more. I almost felt like they resented me for not being a Christian the majority of my life like they had. I could be wrong, but this is the impression they gave out. I'm not sure I would want to have been Christian my whole life. I've learnt so many valuable lessons now through living a bit of a "fast lifestyle" that I'm not sure if I'd been a Christian my whole life, that my relationship with Jesus would be as strong. I believe I felt his presence in the darkest times of my life. It's through that and that alone that I realized his overwhelming and unconditional love for me. The suffering led to my salvation.

I started to have the common misconception that I was too far gone to become a Christian. Even some of my closest friends used that term when they realized I was looking at different churches.

"You, a Christian? Didn't realize Jesus specialized in time machines," they'd often joke.

I started to believe that this was the case – it was far too late for me to tell myself I was a Christian. My behaviour in the past surely couldn't be that of anyone who would call himself a Christian. That week, I had planned to go to a church in Stratford-upon-Avon, but was starting to talk myself out of it. I began thinking about the other guys my age I had met at various churches and how I could never emulate the behaviour and commitment to God they showed as young men.

"God wants guys like that, not like me," I would say.

I had gone out on a Saturday night with my friends and had got very drunk. I remember coming back home at about three in the morning thinking, *Well, there's no chance I'm going to that church tomorrow now. I'm going to be far too hungover.* I didn't really see myself getting up till gone lunchtime on Sunday – that was always the way when I had a heavy night. To my surprise, I woke up shortly after eight in the morning. I didn't feel hungover, I was fresh and ready to go. I was caught off guard. *Well, there's no excuse now,* I thought to myself.

I got up, had my breakfast and prepared for my visit to this new church. I can remember there being a sense of hope and optimism that morning. I really felt something was pulling me along to go to this church service.

I arrived at the hotel car park where the church service was taking place. I sat in my car, a bit nervous about going in. I felt like this was a defining moment for me, after walking away from the churches I had visited so far. I didn't want to feel like I was walking away from God again. As I sat in my car, I saw many different individuals, couples and families walking into the hotel, presumably for the service. I felt like I wasn't good enough to be around these people who were seemingly perfect. Again, doubts were starting to creep into my head.

"You can never be like these people."

"God doesn't want you."

"You're too far gone."

The sinister voices hissed at me. I must have been wrestling with those thoughts for a good ten minutes in my car. Then I took some deep breaths and cleared my head, reassuring myself that I knew God wanted me to come to this service today.

When I entered the room where the service was taking place, the worship had already begun. I sat on the back row, hoping not to draw any attention to myself, and so I had the option of slipping out of the room quickly if I needed to.

As the worship songs continued, I remember looking around and wondering why all these people seemed to be so happy, even jubilant. I wanted whatever they were drinking, that's for sure! As I continued to look around, I once again was taken aback by an overwhelming presence, an overwhelming sense of unconditional love.

I sat in a row by myself but it felt like someone had walked over to stand next to me and put their hand on my shoulder. When this happened, I felt goosebumps, I felt safe, I felt peace and I felt home. Again, it's such a hard feeling to describe – you just have to feel it. I remember a tear ran down my face. I had been longing to feel like this again ever since my experience when I was attacked, wondering if I ever would again. Now here it was. I didn't even have to question what it was; I knew it was Jesus. I felt like I was in his presence, that he stood right next to me. I remember just repeatedly muttering, "I'm so sorry. I'm really, really sorry." I felt as though I needed to apologize for everything. Tears continued to run down my face. I don't think Jesus was there to hear my apologies, he was there to reassure me I was in the right place and I was loved.

After the worship, a woman preached and, as she spoke, I couldn't believe the words that were coming out of her mouth. All the doubts that I had that week, the worries that God would reject me, the past mistakes that I had made and whether God could forgive them were all addressed in her words.

She said that God doesn't have favourites, that God is greater than our doubts. No matter where we may be in our lives or what we have done in the past, God will always accept us if we trust in Him to save us. God loves each and every single one of us. Word for word she was addressing all of the thoughts and questions I had been asking myself that week. I felt like there was a presence to make sure I listened to every one of her words clearly. The message was for me: God wanted to make sure I came to that church to listen to this message and feel that sense of peace again. I was overcome with emotion and was desperately trying to hold all of that in.

As the service drew to a close, I think someone saw that I was looking quite overwhelmed. He approached and introduced himself as Steve, and I felt so relaxed with him that I was soon telling him about me, what brought me to church that day and how the message that I just heard was something I felt God really wanted me to listen to. He introduced to me to a couple of people at the church. Everyone I met seemed so friendly, I almost wondered what the catch was. It didn't seem normal to me for these people to have genuine interest and care in getting to know a complete stranger. I was then introduced to the church leader, who gave me a warm embrace, welcoming me to the church. Then he said a prayer over me. It was a defining moment. It was so foreign to me to feel love from a complete stranger. I was able to pass my worries, cares, anxiety, depression and past mistakes onto God. As I closed my eyes, listening to the prayer, I could hear God telling me to let things go and give them to Him. It's as if He was there with open arms, ready for me to pass over all my past troubles and mistakes.

I know that this was the church where I could mark a new beginning. I felt reborn and forgiven and, since that day, I know Jesus as my Lord and saviour.

CHAPTER 24

Since becoming a Christian, I've dealt with a few questions that I've always found a bit baffling, especially from my friends. I think maybe there're some misconceptions about Christians and their views, especially when I get asked some of the following questions.

1. Since you're a Christian now, do you hate gay people?

Absolutely not. From my background of working in different entertainment industries, a lot of my close friends are gay. In fact, one of my best friends told me only recently that he was gay. I was the first person he came out to. Some of the greatest creative minds I've had the pleasure of meeting are homosexual.

I don't think as a Christian I could ever judge a homosexual. In my life I have lied, slept around, had a bad relationship with alcohol and been selfish. I have no right to judge anyone. I leave that up to God.

Jesus says, "A new command I give you: Love one another. As I have loved you, so you must love one another. By this everyone will know that you are my disciples, if you love one another." (John 13:34,35)

I don't think any true Christians hold any hatred for homosexuals at all. Jesus doesn't hate. Do I think a homosexual would go to the gates of heaven and be told, "Sorry, no gays allowed"? No. The most important thing we can do is know who Jesus is and have a relationship with him.

I feel that this is a question that Christians get a bit of a hard time on, but it is an important question, not least because there are some who openly disapprove. I remember recently walking through a Gay Pride event in London and seeing a group of people protesting against the event. There were signs saying, "God hates fags", "Homos in hell", "Repent or perish". I remember asking myself what Jesus would do in this situation. I don't believe that the Jesus who I know would ever be protesting with those people. But I don't believe they are full of hate; I believe they are honouring the word of God in the Bible as it's written.

I'd be dishonest if I said that this question doesn't worry me, and I'd be lying if I said I will be out there waving the Gay Pride flag, but the Bible teaches us to love even those we disagree with. Never hate. God is the ultimate judge.

2. Do you think anyone who isn't a Christian is going to hell?

Thankfully, that's not my call. As a Christian, I would just trust in God's judgement. I believe God knows all of our hearts and thoughts. When our life is over, I don't believe you end up somewhere for eternity on a technicality. God isn't going to say, "You know, I really wish I could let you in but my hands are tied. There's nothing I can do." God knows us all better than we know ourselves, and his judgement on us all will be the right one.

3 Don't Christians think suicides go to hell?

I really struggle with answering this. It hurts me that some Christians may feel like this is the case. But again, I trust in God's judgement. I would struggle to see how God would send someone who took their own life to hell, especially if they knew Jesus.

It irks me a bit when people say Christians can't be depressed if they truly know the joy of the Lord. This is something I completely disagree with. If you look in the Bible, you can see that followers of God do not only experience positive emotions. You can look at quotations about feeling sorrow and restless.

"My soul is bereft of peace; I've forgotten what happiness is." (Lamentations 3:17–19)

Negative emotions are necessary to the Christian experience.

Jesus Himself experienced low emotions, such as when he was weeping in the garden of Gethsemane. No one said to Him then, "Jesus, why are you reacting this way? Don't you trust God?"

We live in a broken world. Depression can be the impact of seeing that this world is not how it's supposed to be. Christians shouldn't feel guilty for having depressed feelings. It shouldn't be seen as a "wrong emotion" and certainly doesn't mean you don't believe in the joy of the Lord. Joy isn't a replacement for depressive feelings in the Christian experience. Life is not either total joy or total depression. The joy is the belief that God is going to fix this broken world. He will usher in a world where there is no sorrow, no crying, no pain and no death anymore. Joy can streak its way through depression but it does not replace it.

Personally, if I'm asked whether a person who decided to take their own life is in hell, my answer would always be no. We're not saved based on the last thing that we do. We're saved by the grace and mercy of God. Those who commit suicide are in a place of deep, deep anguish, distress, hopelessness, pain and mental illness. We ought to view that with compassion. We can't blame someone who takes their own life, we can't be angry at that person and feel we can say they are out of reach of God's grace. The Lord does not persecute suicides; mental health issues such as depression are an illness. When you're living in a sick, dark world, it is understandable to feel as though you can't take it anymore, that there's no way out and you're too tired to carry on. We are in no place to judge anyone whose demons are taking over their lives.

4   Where do you stand on assisted suicide?

There's also the question where Christians may stand with assisted suicide or "death with dignity", as some people refer to it. It's a really taboo issue and, to be honest, I have no idea what the right or wrong answer is. Personally, I try to think of people's personal circumstances, how much pain they may be in and what the future holds for them. I can't say for sure if I had completely lost the function of my limbs or was dying from a terminal illness whether the relief and temptation of dying with dignity might seem appealing. I think for me, the biggest fear for me as I grow old would be the thought of losing my mind. I think if I was ever going to suffer with any type of dementia, losing all sense of my character, creativity, memories and recognition of loved ones, I personally would want to end my life before that happened, not just for myself but for the sake of my loved ones. So, in some cases I can completely understand why people take that decision. But it would certainly be a drastic choice to make.

On this topic, however, I was horrified with a documentary I watched recently. It was about a 24-year-old female in Belgium who had been approved for assisted suicide via lethal injection. She had no physical health problems but felt like she had enough of being depressed. She went through a process and met with doctors about the procedure, but I was so shocked that she was approved as someone who, at that age, could make the decision that she was going to die. The documentary followed the girl over a one-year process, adamant throughout that she wanted to die. On the day of her scheduled death, only a couple of hours before the injection was to take place, she changed her mind and pulled out of the entire procedure. Surely, this in itself shows there is a massive problem with that law in Belgium. Assisted suicide should absolutely not be used in that way.

5 Why does God let so much suffering happen in the world?

Again, it's a fair enough question and I don't have a magic answer. It's a question I've wrestled with myself. Why do we suffer when it's not our fault? What is the purpose of suffering? We don't choose it and it doesn't allow us to grow or gain in any way. It's a terrible thing. But we all experience it and we all have to endure it.

Why would a loving, kind God allow that to happen? The only way I can get my head around it is that I believe that God isn't the cause of suffering. We are the cause of suffering. Suffering is man-made. When we think of war, murder, rape, lies and cheating, these all come back to us as humans. I understand that this doesn't apply to all suffering, there's some that is beyond anyone's control: an earthquake, illness and so many injustices. It's something I ask myself from time to time. But I believe it's God exposing to us that things aren't how they should be on this planet, that the ultimate cause is sin. Adam and Eve rebelled against God and by doing so cursed the earth. I don't believe God intended there to be a world where there was sickness, pain and death but we broke God's commandments. We've broken every one of them. I believe the more we rebel and the more we defy Him, the more we see this plague of suffering coming into the world. It looms over humanity and overwhelms us.

Why doesn't God just come down and sort all this mess out? Well, my answer would be that He's leaving us in this world of suffering to give us time to accept Jesus as our saviour.

6   What stops people believing in Jesus?

I know a lot of people who want to believe in God and want to know Jesus but feel like some of these issues push them away from accepting Him. I feel this is where Christians and non-believers need to discuss these views more, in a healthy way. I totally get that people are very passionate about their views and beliefs, but as someone who became a Christian in his late 20s, I feel it's okay to have healthy discussions with Christians about the aspects of faith we may each struggle to get our heads around. As a Christian, I believe we need to understand that people have difficult questions or doubts that they feel need addressing. I like to think most Christians are more than happy to discuss these topics in a constructive way.

Becoming a Christian was a huge change for me. Some of my friends resented and teased me for it as I changed my lifestyle and changed my priorities. But as hard as it has been to make that transition, it's something that I would not change for the world. I am at peace with myself, and having that peace in my life is priceless. I was looking in all the wrong places in this secular world to find happiness, but God was able to offer something even better and that was peace. I understand why my lifelong friends found my transition into Christianity hard. I didn't show interest in getting drunk anymore, going to nightclubs, strip clubs or on the lads' holidays. As much as I felt my friends resented my faith, they all still did show their support by coming to my baptism in 2019. It's just a shame I've also had to deal with lots of offensive jokes, voicemails, discussions and images about my faith. But I guess we've got to take the rough with the smooth! Of course, I love and forgive my friends. I've certainly sent my fair share of banter their way too.

I don't know if you know Jesus, and I'm not going to plead with you to accept Him. It has to be a personal decision. I had to experience the Holy Spirit for me to pursue a relationship with Jesus. But if you're longing for that sense of peace like I was, trust me, it's certainly worth looking into more. I can't express to you enough how much finding peace gave me. The more I think about it, I just can't believe we are here by accident. To me that notion is madness. Science is wonderful and explains so much for us, but when it comes to the really big questions, it can never explain why. I don't believe when we die, that's it, that's a wrap. There just has to be more to it.

CHAPTER 25

What does it take to be happy? We have a story in our head about how life is supposed to be. Somebody's story might be that you work hard at school, you're a nice person and then you grow up, take care of yourself, fall in love, have beautiful children and live happily ever after. Someone else's story might be to work really hard, get a degree, work for a big company, climb up through the ranks until you're the chairman of the company and you become wealthy, successful and respected in your life. Whatever your story in your head is, there are striking similarities. People feel to be happy and complete in their life that they have to achieve an enormous amount. We live in a culture where we teach people that we're not enough unless we do something special or unique.

We define those things in interesting ways. Being a parent is not special or unique, we don't treat teachers or nurses as special or unique and we don't pay them accordingly for the huge responsibilities they have. Yet footballers are worshipped and paid astronomical amounts. It's a messed-up way of life that we've created.

Why is there so much depression in society today? Why are suicides skyrocketing in the Western world? The simple answer is because of us. The culture we are creating, especially for young people, isn't a healthy one.

We need to focus on the beauty and joy around us. We need to love each other; we need to bond again.

Yes, there are biological reasons why people may get depressed. It can be due to a naturally low level of serotonin in the brain, and there are drugs that will help take care of it. But I don't believe the drugs are the answer long-term. The longer I dealt with depression, the more I felt there must be more to it. I felt that taking drugs to treat depression is like putting on a coat when it rains: it won't stop the rain from falling, it just means that for a short while you don't get drenched.

And if the only cause of depression and anxiety was a chemical imbalance, why are the levels rising so quickly? It just didn't seem right to me. As I researched depression more and spent time praying about it, I felt that the causes are mostly not in our heads, but as a result of the way we are living.

When you look at it that way, a different solution arises. Sometimes, people just feel alone. Feeling like you can't reach out to people, feeling like you're dealing with this all by yourself and not wanting to burden loved ones with it causes the incredible sense of pain that loneliness gives you. Our instincts as humans should be to tribe together, but now we live in a society where we disband and live alone, feeling like we can deal with things ourselves. I believe that loneliness is a significant factor in why we are seeing depression and suicide rates rising. We need to meet in groups, trying out new activities where we can meet new people and communicate.

It's something I worry about with our children today. Kids don't go outside, play and bond like they used to. Now they would much rather spend their time looking at a screen rather than their friend's face. The more we overexpose young children to technology, the more we are imprisoning them. There is a British study that found that the average British child now spends less time outdoors than an inmate in prison. That's a really worrying statistic. We neglect the most important things in life at our peril. And you are not going to find any of those things on the internet; that's something even Amazon doesn't stock.

Do you remember the last time you had fun in your life? Do you remember when things felt easy and life flowed along? As we grow up, we lose sight of how amazing life can be because we feel burdened by responsibilities and the expectations and pressures of modern-day life. Reconnect with what you love to do. Make a commitment to do that and watch your life change for the better. It doesn't matter what anyone else may think as long as you are not hurting anyone. Only you can measure your own happiness.

Depression robs us of the things we love: our peace and joy. If you're facing the battle with depression today, believe me, I know what you're going through: countless hours churning over your mistakes and inadequacies.

There are some things in life that are out of our control and we can't change them, however much we might want to. The choice that we have, though, is to either give up or keep on going. What are you going to believe? Are you going to believe in yourself or are you going to believe people's judgement of you? Are you going to believe people when they say you're a failure? That no one really likes you and no one really cares about you? No. Trust yourself.

And be honest with those around you. When people ask you how you are, and you say, "Fine," why would they not believe you are fine? If you don't tell them, they won't know. Be prepared to be vulnerable. Let them see the depression, the pain, the anxiety, the fear and all things that you're going through. Then they can support you and you will come out the other side of as a stronger version of yourself.

There's a saying, "You always find something in the last place you look." Of course you do, because you don't stop looking until you find it. When you fall down you may feel you don't have the strength to get up again, but if you keep trying there's always hope that you will. It's only the end when you give up.

It's time to get up. It's time to fight back. Getting up might mean going to see a doctor, attending counselling, starting medication, going to work, stopping binge drinking or even just deciding you are not going to let your life be controlled by depression.

Get started. It won't be easy; at times, it will be really hard. But you are not alone. These challenges that you face are going to do their best to take you down. Do not let them. Fight them.

You might be going through hell and I know how difficult it can be. I have been in the valley of darkness; I know how bleak things can be. But I also know this: it's always too soon to quit. You've got to believe your best days are in front of you. You've got to believe that your future is brighter than your past and you've got to believe that the best is yet to come.

If you're in a dark place today, I plead with you. Reach out to your loved ones, reach out to God, pray, go and see a doctor, exercise and get outside. Use your pain as your tool for your greatest growth.

Find your purpose. It's okay to not be okay. It's just not okay to stay that way.

CHAPTER 26

In 2019, I was sitting on a bench by the river in Stratford-upon-Avon. It was a beautiful summer evening, with a light, refreshing breeze. I remember sitting there as someone who felt reborn, who felt at peace and someone who was no longer a slave to depression.

I hope I'm on the right path, I remember thinking to myself. My friends were struggling with my faith in God and didn't understand why I wanted to change my lifestyle so much. To them it was almost as though I was a different person – they may have argued a more boring person. One of my closest friends even asked me if I had considered that I was perhaps being brainwashed by the church. Yeah, some of the comments bothered me, but nothing could take away that sense of peace I was feeling and I wouldn't give that up for anything. I sat on that bench, hoping I was now on the right path, wondering if I was through the worst with my battle with depression and wondering what the future held for me.

As I was thinking about these things, a shabby-looking man was walking past me. He was probably in his 60s, his clothes looked tattered and worn, he had a very messy, long beard, but although his appearance seemed rather grotty, his demeanour was quite the opposite. He had a spring in his step and just so happened to be whistling my favourite song, "Smile" by Nat King Cole – I couldn't help but smile to myself.

"Evening friend," the man waved at me.

"Evening," I replied. "Lovely one, isn't it?"

"You from around here?" he asked.

"Nah, about half an hour away, I just love it here," I replied.

"It's the simple things in life, eh?" he chuckled as I smiled back.

He started to approach and before I knew it he was sitting beside me on the bench. I have to say I was a bit reluctant for him to sit next to me. I wasn't really in the mood to chat, and he had an uncertain, not-so-pleasant stench to him.

"Why don't you move out here if you love it here so much?" he asked.

"Just not sure if it's the right time at the moment. Lots going on," I said.

"I see," he replied back bluntly, before adding, "Just be sure not to overthink it too much. That's all people do these days, overthink. When their gut gives them a reason to do something their head gives them three reasons not to. It's never wrong to go with your heart," he insisted.

"Yeah," I answered back. I felt like I was humouring him at this stage. I was trying to think of a swift excuse to leave.

"We all have lots going on," he said, "Sometimes things overwhelm us, especially for you youngsters. I don't envy your generation at all. Things used to be so much simpler. Whatever's going on, we all have the strength to push through it – that's if we want to. But sadly, we live in a world where doubt is overcoming faith. You know what I would say to you youngsters?" he said.

"No," I answered and thought, *but I bet you're going to tell me.*

"I would say, you have the opportunity to show the world what you're really made of. Don't let doubts suppress you. Don't focus on the doubts. There is within you a spirit that is greater than whatever is going on around you. Doubts will only stop you from taking the form of who you're supposed to be."

At that point those words struck something in me. It was almost an awakening as I saw how my doubts and regrets had been taking over my life. What was I getting out of it by putting myself through that torment? Nothing.

"Anyway, sorry I've gone on. I'll leave you to it. I hope your path brings you to town soon," he smiled. "Take care, Lawrence," he said before strolling away.

I never did see that gentleman again. I hope that one day I do. His words are something I will never forget. Since that moment, I have now been baptized and accepted Jesus as my Lord and saviour and I am trying to learn more and more about Him each day. Trying to ask myself, "What would Jesus do?" in certain situations has really lifted me up higher than I've ever been. I have written a few children's books, which has been an amazing experience for me. I've travelled all around the UK to different schools, libraries and events to encourage children to read books, and I've adopted my little rescue dog, Robin. No prizes for guessing who I named him after.

But the greatest thing I have in my life right now is peace. I have peace within myself and I urge everyone to do what it takes to find that within yourself, especially if you're struggling. You may have to make sacrifices, cut back and strip things away that seem impossible, such as binge drinking, social media and the need to be liked by everyone. But I promise you, during that difficult journey, when you find peace within yourself, it's the most wonderful thing you could ever hope for.

I owe that man on the bench a lot. His words helped me flush the doubts away. There is still one thing, however, that baffles me to this day: How the fuck did he know my name?

ABOUT CHERISH EDITIONS

Cherish Editions is a bespoke self-publishing service for authors of mental health, wellbeing and inspirational books.

As a division of Trigger Publishing, the UK's leading independent mental health and wellbeing publisher, we are experienced in creating and selling positive, responsible, important and inspirational books, which work to destigmatize the issues around mental health and improve the mental health and wellbeing of those who read our titles.

Founded by Adam Shaw, a mental health advocate, author and philanthropist, and leading psychologist Lauren Callaghan, Cherish Editions aims to publish books that provide advice, support and inspiration. We nurture our authors so that their stories can unfurl on the page, helping them to share their uplifting and moving stories.

Cherish Editions is unique in that a percentage of the profits from the sale of our books goes directly to leading mental health charity Shaw Mind, to deliver its vision to provide support for those experiencing mental ill health.

Find out more about Cherish Editions by visiting cherisheditions.com or by joining us on:
Twitter @cherisheditions
Facebook @cherisheditions
Instagram @cherisheditions

Cherish
EDITIONS

ABOUT SHAWMIND

A proportion of profits from the sale of all Trigger books go to their sister charity, Shawmind, also founded by Adam Shaw and Lauren Callaghan. The charity aims to ensure that everyone has access to mental health resources whenever they need them.

You can find out more about the work Shawmind do by visiting their website shawmind.org or joining them on:

Twitter @Shaw_Mind
Facebook @ShawmindUK
Instagram @Shaw_Mind

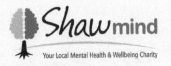

Your Local Mental Health & Wellbeing Charity